Childless Couples

Childless Couples

Social Consequences of Sterility and Infertility

Vinita Lavania

RAWAT PUBLICATIONS

Jaipur • New Delhi • Bangalore • Mumbai • Hyderabad

ISBN 81-316-0013-0

The publication of this book was financially supported by ICSSR and the responsibility for the facts stated, opinions expressed or conclusions reached, is entirely that of the author and that ICSSR accepts no responsibility for them.

ICSSR Consultant
Prof. N. Jayaram

Published by
Prem Rawat for **Rawat Publications**
Satyam Apts., Sector 3, Jawahar Nagar, Jaipur 302 004 (India)
Phone: 0141 265 1748 / 7006 Fax: 0141 265 1748
E-mail: info@rawatbooks.com
Website: www.rawatbooks.com

New Delhi Office
4858/24, Ansari Road, Daryaganj, New Delhi 110 002
Phone: 011-23263290

Also at Bangalore, Mumbai and Hyderabad

Typeset by Rawat Computers, Jaipur
Printed at Nice Printing Press, New Delhi

In memory of

Prof. B.K. Lavania

Contents

Foreword

The present research study is an attempt to explore the social consequences related to the issue of childlessness. Since childlessness is a problem that affects the couple, the family and the community at large, an effort has been made to look at this problem in a holistic manner.

In Indian society, a childless woman is considered as *'Banjh'* or 'dry womb'. Her sterility or *'barrenness' is* a stigma for her. Woman who cannot give her family an heir is seen as a curse. Her life will always be seen as incomplete due to her lack of motherhood. Due to her own sterility or her husband's sterility, she is not considered worthy to attend family, religious or social functions as her presence in such occasions is considered inauspicious.

In past few years several studies have been conducted by medical and social scientists in the field of sterility and infertility. Their work is mainly based on biological and psychological aspects of sterility and infertility. By contrast there is little work on the social and cultural aspects of childlessness. This book hopes to address this lacuna in the literature by exploring this issue from an organic as well as social and psychological perspective. The social institutional dimension of childless couples is prominently determined by the caste considerations, duration of marital life, occupation, rural-urban residence and type of social class. Through a combination of qualitative and quantitative methods, these factors have been taken into consideration to provide a complete picture of the situation of the childless couples in India. It is also felt that this research can be used to provide practical solutions to the problem faced by such couples.

The change in the life of the childless couples can be brought about only by change in social traditions and social institutional interactions. It requires change in perception and attitude of the community by removal of social stigma attached with the childless couples, especially women. The change can be brought about only when childlessness is considered as physical, not social disability. Thus, modern values could, perhaps mitigate the agonies of childless couples.

Dr. Vinita Lavania has examined the difficult problem from a number of different angles and with great sensitivity. She has done commendable job by addressing emerging issues of childless couples in a transforming society. Such work represents the innovativeness in a new generation of sociologist, who are engaged in many of India's social problems and doing justice both to India's tradition and her modern ambitions. The book will be valuable for the readers in sociology of family, social work and social welfare agencies.

Udaipur **Mohan Advani**
15 October 2005

Preface

It is said that there is happiness in this world because children keep getting born. Conversely, absence of children can result in considerable unhappiness as well, especially in the traditional patriarchal Indian society with its inexplicable emphasis on a male child, if infertility or sterility causes such an absence. Moreover, very often, it is the childless women who are stigmatised and who bear the brunt of social wrath, that ranges from sarcastic, caustic remarks to being ostracised, even if it is their husbands who are responsible for the childlessness. The net result of this situation is a simmering turbulence (among the childless couple, and especially in the wife), that engulfs the entire Indian society with its adverse effects.

Thus, after defining sterility and infertility, this study traces the causes of childlessness (which may be due to organic problems, or psychological factors or lack of proper knowledge). Besides, it also seeks to analyse the socio-cultural aspects associated with childlessness. This study, based on eight closely-linked hypotheses, lays special emphasis on the societal attitude towards childlessness, the changes in interpersonal relationships within and outside the family, and the subsequent negative behavioural changes that occur between the aggrieved couple itself.

The methodology adopted for this study includes a research design, which is adequately suited for the 120 infertile and 120 sterile couples, from Rajasthan. The methodology also covers tools like interview schedules, field-observations, and case studies, and the quantitative data collected from these tools has been interpreted through some of the latest statistical methods. Since one of the objectives of this study is also to identify and implement methods to mitigate tensions caused by childlessness, information was sought from respondents on how they managed such tensions.

The various remedial measures, including different kinds of medical interference and alternative therapies, which can handle a gamut of problems associated with childlessness, have also been taken up in considerable detail. Adoption of children has also been discussed as an important alternative for confirmed cases of sterility and infertility. All these measures finally aim at minimising the adverse effects of childlessness, both at personal and social levels.

Considerable work has already been undertaken on this subject, and more is likely to follow. This study is an attempt to highlight the contemporary aspects of sterility and infertility in India; identify their social consequences; and enumerate some of the technology-backed remedies. All these together, one hopes, will overcome the ill effects of childlessness on a society with an otherwise better level of awareness.

Vinita Lavania

৫৩৪০

Acknowledgements

Without the help of many persons and organisations, this research would never have been completed and certainly not in a timely and professional manner.

First and foremost, I would like to thank Dr. Mohan Advani, former Professor of Sociology, Mohanlal Sukhadia University, Udaipur, who has guided me through all phases of work on this project. I cannot forget to express my level of indebtedness to him, my Ph.D advisor as well as a family friend.

I am also profoundly grateful to Dr. Y.S. Jhala, Principal, Bhupal Nobles' P.G. College, Udaipur, whose guidance and encouragement have been a constant source of inspiration for me. Dr. Chakrapani Upadhyay and Dr. Arun Zachariah, two colleagues from B.N.P.G. College have also provided so much encouragement, support and critical feedback on my work. I wish to put gratitude for them.

Dr. Balveer Singh and Dr. Monika Nagori have also provided me many necessary resources to complete my research and I express my thanks to them.

Since my research project is closely linked with human health, I received much counsel from specialists in the medical profession – My thanks go to Dr. A.S. Gupta, Dr. K.R. Sharma, Dr. Ajay Murdia, Dr. Satish Shrimali, Dr. Kalpana Upmanyu as well as to many other eminent medical luminaries for their professional guidance.

I am grateful to Indian Council of Social Science Research, New Delhi for awarding me a grant, that made this book's publication possible. I am also grateful to Prof. N. Jayaram, Professor, Tata Institute of Social Sciences, Mumbai for his help in transforming my dissertation into book form.

Similarly, this study could never have been possible, without the enthusiastic involvement of many infertile couples, who shared their personal details with me and thus provided the bulk of data for this book. I thank these respondents for overcoming the social inhibitions that made communication on a topic of this kind, and for their generous and openhearted cooperation.

My father-in-law, Late Prof. B.K. Lavania has also been an inspiring presence in my life. In his joint role as academic guide and also as caring parent, he has provided me with all the requisite academic inputs and the determination to undertake and complete this work. As such, I dedicate this book to him.

My fond and loving thanks are due to all the other members of my family – especially to my mother-in-law, Mrs. Basant Bala Lavania, Mausi, Ms. Vimlesh Sharma, my husband, Mr. Vivek Lavania, and also to our son, Akshat, and my parents Dr. Mahesh Chandra Sharma and Mrs. Shashi Sharma. Without their constant encouragement and support this project would never have come to fruition.

I would like to acknowledge the numerous other persons and agencies that have directly or indirectly helped in the completion of this research project, who for reason of space go unmentioned here.

And of course thanks go to the editors and staff of Rawat Publications for their constant professionalism – their labour has assumed that this important topic will reach a wide audience.

Finally, I express my devoted thanks to the Almighty for all His blessings on my work and for enabling me to give this shape to my research, which I hope will contribute humbly in making this world a better place.

Vinita Lavania

List of Tables

1

Social Status of Childless Couples

In ancient India, marriage was considered to be necessary for the complete fulfilment of the purpose of life of men and women. Without marriage it was believed that they could not achieve 'moksha'. It is evident from our holy books, old stories and myths, how people were blessed with children after praying and fasting and performing various types of religious rituals. Even today it is seen that some people who believe that they got their child due to some prayers or some incantations, dress him up with clothes from other people for a certain duration of time. They believe that their child will survive by doing so, and their curse of being childless will be washed out.

Marriage is a time honoured, the universal institution, and birth of a child is the climax of happy union, fulfilment of a cherished dream and the ultimate desire of a married couple (Dixit, 1991). Every human being has an instinctive desire to become a parent and look after the offspring. Being a parent has many rewards and pleasures. For most people, to live alone, even with the loving mate, is unthinkable. Parenthood, as a stage of life, is characterised by the need to look after, to take care, to give both materially and in terms of affection. For a woman, it is also an expression of creativity and has both biological and psychological roots (Anand, 1984).

Fecundity, or ability to produce children, has a positive social value. Procreation is socially desirable for religious and family reasons. Children ensure the continuation of the family lineage. Generally, couples who do not bear children within a few years of their marriage, start worrying. Amongst married couples who do not use any contraceptives, about 40 per cent pregnancies occur within first six months and about 80 per cent within one year. Only 5 per cent of such couples do not conceive. These are the probable cases of infertility where medical aid is sought (Sharma, 1990). The inability of the couple, either to conceive or to produce a live birth throughout the marital life, is known as childlessness.

Childlessness has been variously described as a "syndrome of multiple origins, a consequence or manifestation of disease rather than a disease itself, a biological impairment, a psychosomatic disorder, a condition characterising a couple rather than an individual, a failure to conform to cultural prescription, to produce and a failure to fulfil the personal desire to beget a child". The lack of uniform definitions has hounded research on childlessness while it is clear that infertility, childlessness or sterility all refer to the inability of a couple to conceive or bear a child when desired (Jejeebhoy, 1998).

Sterility is the total inability to reproduce. It means inability to produce an offspring and it is the state of being free from living micro-organisms' asepsis. Sterility is due to a condition that cannot be corrected (*Churchill's Medical Dictionary*, 1981). Sterility is the state or quality of being sterile that means incapable of producing others of its kind; barren or deprived of its usual power of function; ineffective. Sterility is inability to reproduce sexually. It causes in humans glandular imbalance, disease and psychological problems (*Collin's Concise Encyclopaedia*, 1984).

Sterility is the condition of being infertile by reason of failure to conceive or reproduce the species—in general, the inability to produce progeny, both male and female, the state of being aseptic or free from all living micro-organisms and their spores (*Butterworth's Medical Dictionary*, 1990). Infertility is failure to conceive and produce a child. It is slightly different from the term 'sterility' which is inability to conceive and produce a child, where, after all the necessary investigation it has been confirmed that conception is not possible. Medically, and most precisely we can say that infertility is the failure of the unification of the egg and the sperm, which ultimately results in the birth of a child. *The Penguin Dictionary of Psychology* defines infertility as, "the condition of having no offspring, which is temporary or reversible". In medical terminology, "infertility is an inability in a woman to conceive or in a man to induce conception" (Martin, 1987). World Health Organisation (WHO) defines it, "as a failure to conceive despite two years of cohabitation and exposure to pregnancy" (WHO, 1991). Infertility is involuntary childlessness. According to the standard medical definition, a woman will be diagnosed as infertile when the woman does not become pregnant after a year of intercourse without contraception. It is not just a woman's disease. Infertility is a couple's problem (Harrison, 1964). The actual definition of infertility is somewhat elastic; the classical period of time is usually taken two years after a healthy marriage, without any contraception. But, in well over half the patients attending an infertility clinic for the first time, the period of infertility, is shorter than this. The relative speed with which the investigations are carried out can be slightly flexible, depending upon both, the age of the patient and the duration of the condition.

As WHO (1991) defines, it is clear that infertility, childlessness or sterility all refer to the inability of couples to conceive or bear children when desired. Yet, there tends to be some variation in the specific definitions adopted by clinicians, demographers and other researchers. Variation occurs largely in (a) the reference period used to establish infertility; and (b) in the classification of women who have experienced pregnancy but not a live birth.

Infertility in human beings is the inability of a woman to conceive or of a man to father children. Both the man and the woman may be able to produce with a different partner. For this reason, infertility is usually regarded as a condition pertaining to two people as a couple, rather than as individuals. Infertility may be temporary and treatable or it may be permanent. Permanent infertility is called sterility. A couple with repeated miscarriages is also considered to be infertile.

Infertility can be primary, if the couple has never conceived despite cohabitation and exposure to pregnancy (not contraception) for a period of two years. Primary infertility is also referred to as primary sterility.

Infertility can be secondary, if a couple fails to conceive following a previous pregnancy, despite cohabitation and exposure to pregnancy (in the absence of contraceptives, breast-feeding or post partum amenorrhoea) for a period of two years. This is also known as secondary sterility.

Infertility is a severe threat to masculinity and femininity, which leads to aggression, depression and emotional complication. There is an unspoken fear of loss of significant relationship, because both, man and woman are hurt, tired and under great pressure; they feel depleted of physical and emotional energy. They may become less able to fulfil each other's need and thereby suffer a loss of closeness, to the point of feeling worlds apart (Mazor, 1979). Another supporting survey of White and David (1977) concluded that the infertile individuals might undergo a loss of relationship, health, status, prestige, self-esteem, self-confidence, security, fantasy and loss of something or someone of great symbolic value. According to Gupta and Shrivastava (1982), the wives are more emotionally disturbed as compared to their husbands. Sometimes relatives and friends did not give genuine support, according to majority of the couples. Pregnant women and other people's children often evoked negative feelings among them. Lalos et al., (1985) observed that the infertile women are depressed, isolated and they feel guilty. There was no balance in the life of the couples. There was hope one week and grief the next. This resulted in depression, anger and guilt. Infertile women exhibited various psychosexual maladjustment because infertility itself may provoke emotional problems, rather than serve as the result. Abse and Sandler (1966) identified the increased frequency of committing suicide by the childless couples, and this shows the degree of stress in them.

Shapiro and Constance (1982) concluded that infertility affects the marital relationships on the aspects such as sexual identity, self-esteem, communication patterns and future life choices. According to Polumbo and Kraft (1980), the negative influence on sexual life was most pronounced among the infertile women because they felt responsible for childlessness. It was also observed by Jacobson and Lalos (1985) that infertile couples undergo grief, depression, guilt and feelings of inferiority and isolation; women openly admitted more symptoms than their partners because infertility was found in them, and marital relationships and sexual life were also affected. On the other hand, Adler (1985) reported that the infertile men who scored high on masculinity were often associated with fewer problems of coping, specifically in terms of their self-esteem, body image, marital adjustment, psychiatric symptoms and self-defeating behaviour.

Infertility imposes a strain on any marriage when the basic human need of parenthood is frustrated. The analysis of impotent cases showed overall constriction in productivity, inability to withstand provoking situations and conflict in the sexual area (White and David, 1977).

Danbick and Judith (1987) reported that the infertility investigation was most stressful for the subjects at the time of initial medical interview, and that the distress was greater for those who themselves identified as having an organic fertility problem. Other factors observed by Bell (1981) were that among a number of infertile patients with different types of disorders, there were some with significant emotional disturbance, some showed evidence of impaired social adjustment, a few reported sexual dysfunction secondary to their infertility and the others showed a deterioration of the marital relationship. Slade and Pauline (1981) also reported that there was no overall significant difference in social role attitudes, but the infertile group showed a significantly more limited range of opinion. They also reported a tendency towards more restrictive sexual attitudes and a high level of guilt feelings.

It was found that infertility had a far more negative influence on the female subjects' behaviour with disappointment, jealousy and marital dissatisfaction. Psychological acceptance of this condition also developed significantly slower in the female group (Brand, 1981). However, Rosenfeld (1984) found that a woman feels inadequate when she fails at the most critical times. Social interrogations as 'hows' and 'whys' make the woman feel tense and it reminds her every now and then that she has failed to conceive. According to Miall (1986), perception of childless women revealed it to be a negative or discreditable attribute. The physically infertile women feel more stigmas, but women with infertile husbands control the information more in order to protect the spouse. Consequently, the wives had a significantly lower level of satisfaction with life than their husbands and there were significant relationships between the spouses for both, marital and sexual satisfaction. It was also found that the divorce rates among infertile marriages were greater than those couples with children or even with a single child—divorce rates were found to be higher in the urban areas as compared to the rural ones (Sharma, 1999).

In contrast, Van Keep and Smith (1975) observed that most of the childless couples had a favourable attitude to other people's children and they like being in their company. Study of Allison and Janet (1979) shows that the role conceptions of infertile groups were significantly more traditional, they reported less role conflict of various kinds and they showed greater occupational commitment. They did not differ significantly on degree of wife-husband role discrepancy or mother's occupational commitment.

THIS STUDY

Childlessness is a problem, which affects the couple, the family and the community at large. An effort has been made to look at this issue in a holistic manner, so that suitable measures of intervention for the management of problem of childlessness could be suggested. The main objectives of the present study are:

1. To study the background characteristics, role and status of the childless couples in society.
2. To explore the nature and types of relationship of childless couples and to study the behavioural patterns of the family, neighbourhood, kinship and community towards childless couples.
3. To analyse the traditional beliefs, norms, values and religious practices related to sterility and infertility.
4. To analyse social and cultural milieu of childless couples in seeking medical assistance and treatment for reproduction.
5. To study tension management processes adopted by the childless couples.
6. To analyse the social consequences of sterility and infertility.

SIGNIFICANCE OF THE STUDY

In past few years several studies have been conducted by medical and social scientists in the field of sterility and infertility—their work is mainly based on biological and psychological aspects of sterility and infertility. There is little work on social and cultural aspects of sterility and infertility, taking into consideration its multifaceted nature. It has been mostly understood and handled as a medical problem, overlooking the personal, social and psychological aspects.

Since ancient times, much importance is being attached to the aspect of infertility. This is evident from our holy books, old stories and myths. It is human nature that the couples desire to have children. Parenthood is related to the 'giving' aspect of love. Among the childless couples this deep-rooted desire is shattered, giving rise to different sorts of problems.

There is one more reason considered necessary for a male-child. Procreation is socially desirable for religious and family reasons, as it is the offspring who is responsible for the continuation of the family line and for performing the last rites and rituals of the parents, for their so-called 'moksha'.

The present study attempts to realise the social consequences of sterility and infertility with social dimensions, and management of the resultant tensions. The study is very important, particularly when the level of modernity and medical health facilities has increased, and yet the social environment plays an important role in shaping the social status of childless couples. Today's generation is educated and career oriented and sometimes young couples plan to enjoy their life for few years after marriage or they want to settle properly. So, they delay their first pregnancy. This type of childlessness is voluntary childlessness and not included in this study.

CAUSES OF CHILDLESSNESS

Many conditions are known to cause or to contribute to infertility. Contrary to the popular belief that infertility is due to some problem in the woman, when studied scientifically, the causes of infertility may be found in both men and women. Broadly speaking, they can be classified as follows (Anand, 1984):

Organic Factors

Factors in Males

(a) *Sex problems*: Some sex problems like premature ejaculation or lack of ejaculation, low sperm counts are directly related to conception when a perfectly fertile man may not be able to reproduce.

(b) *Duct blockage*: If the passage (reproductive tract) between the penis and testes is blocked, there will be no sperms in the semen (azoospermia).

(c) *Hormonal imbalance*: Hormonal imbalance in males can also lead to infertility. Hormonal imbalance can arise due to head injuries, tumours in pituitary or adrenal gland, malfunctioning of pituitary gland, cirrhosis of liver or a thyroid problem.

(d) *Substance abuse*: Excessive use of substances like alcohol, tobacco or drug abuse can create malformed sperms or sperms with poor motility.

(e) *Infections and venereal diseases*: Infections and venereal diseases like Tuberculosis, Gonorrhoea, Chlamydia, Syphilis and other sexually transmitted diseases can also infect male genital tract.

(f) *Medication and its effects*: Some medication can play havoc with the sperm count or with the sex drive. Drugs used for high blood pressure, urinary infections, antibiotics, steroids, etc., have adverse effect on fertility.

Factors in Females

(a) *Tubule obstructions:* In females the leading cause of infertility is tubule obstruction which can result from venereal diseases and pelvic inflammatory diseases.

(b) *Ovulatory problems:* Some women experience ovulatory problems. For example, they may have irregular menstrual cycle, amenorrhoea (absence of menstrual cycle) or an ovulation (failure of the ovaries to release ova or eggs).

(c) *Absence of reproductive organs:* In some women, there may be an absence of one or more reproductive organs.
(d) *Polycystiovarian diseases:* In this case, the females have small multiple cysts in their ovaries. These cysts occur when the regular changes of a normal menstrual cycle are disturbed.
(e) *Endometriosis:* It occurs when the normal endometrial tissue (lining of the uterus) grows outside the uterus.
(f) *Ectopic pregnancy:* Ectopic pregnancy is one, which develops outside the uterus. Most ectopics are found in the fallopian tubes.

Psychological Factors

Problems pertaining to potency always have to do with fear of letting go and losing control, as well as fear of repressed psychological contents. The necessary energy is kept in the head instead of going to where it is needed. There would often be feelings of sexual pressure and tension, as well as of guilt, and some could even feel some spite against an earlier partner. It is not surprising that everything goes wrong. Once you have become more conscious of these things you will realise that it is necessary to go more into your feelings, because sex has nothing to do with intellect (Baginski and Sharamon, 1999).

Emotional stress has been reported to be responsible for the quality and number of sperms in males. Distress and anxiety have been reported as responsible factor for infertility in the females. These factors have an inhibiting effect on psychological process and are therefore responsible for infertility. Certain other psychological factors also result in lack of desire for sex, due to which sexual activity may not be of the required frequency and at the required time and may therefore result in infertility.

Sexual Factors

Sexual factors play a crucial role in infertility directly or indirectly. Infections in genital area, pain during intercourse, lack of satisfaction, lack of desire for sex, etc., are some factors which play an important role for preventing contraception. Any of these conditions may lead to aversion or disinclination for sex and may result in lesser frequency of sex due to which conception may not take place (Anand, 1984).

Sometimes nothing is organically, physiologically, marital and sexually wrong and yet conception does not take place. In such cases, it is found that the couple indulges in intercourse quite often, but not during the fertility period and therefore conception does not take place. In such cases, a little counselling helps to provide the requisite knowledge, which in turn helps in conception (Vaessan, 1984).

Social Circumstantial Factors

Sterility in some women indicates an unconscious rejection of pregnancy, while in others a child is only wanted as a means of binding the partner, indicating an underlying trait of dishonesty. Male sterility indicates fear of close relationship as well of having to bear responsibility for the child (Baginski and Sharamon, 1999).

It has been noted that sometimes all other factors are positive and yet conception does not take place. This may be due to circumstantial factors like the couples staying together but not having enough privacy for sexual union, the frequency of intercourse not being adequate and appropriate, psychological distance in spite of living together, etc. Such problems are reflected among cases that often seek the help of the counsellor, when on medical investigation all tests give positive results and yet conception does not occur. On detailed inquiry, some of the above-mentioned factors are found to be playing a crucial role in failure in conception. Several events, within human control, have been repeatedly identified as causes of the diminished capacity to reproduce. Delayed childbearing has been implicated in the etiology of infertility through the factors of age, which is inversely related to procreative potential. Delayed childbearing has also been linked to use of contraceptives use and abortion that have in turn been tied to ovulatory irregularities, pelvic infections and pelvic adhesions.

It is also seen that certain genetic or social factors seem to be correlated with infertility. Only few researches have been attempted to determine, whether any genetic or social factor correlates with infertility or not. In search for genetic correlates, Mathews and Mathews (1986) found no evidence of an association between genetic inheritance and general human fertility. In contrast, White and David (1977) focussing on infertility in women, found that majority of women came from small families, that 30 per cent had a sister with infertility problems and that 45 per cent had some relative who had trouble in conceiving.

Postan (1990) attempted to determine whether or not any social factor is correlated with infertility and found no consistent linear pattern between childlessness (both voluntary and involuntary) and husband's income or family income. However, he did find a higher incidence of childlessness at both the lower and upper ends of income distribution than in the middle. A study in China observed that infertility was higher in low-income setting in comparison with high-income setting (Mathews and Mathews, 1986). Jejeebhoy (1998) also reported higher incidence of childlessness among lower-income families and attributed them to lack of money for medical procedure.

Regional and Cultural Variations

A multicentric study of infertility conducted by WHO (1994) showed that immediate causes of infertility related to both males and females, and the conditions that directly contribute to infertility vary region-wise and culture-wise. Identifiable factors affecting female infertility include hormonal or endocrine disturbances (menstrual or ovulatory disturbances), tubule factors (cervical or uterine disturbances), sexual dysfunction and congenital abnormalities. The most common were endocrine disturbances (35% globally and 37% in Asia) and tubule factors (32% globally and in Asia). In contrast, sexual dysfunction, congenital abnormalities and acquired non-tubule factors accounted for no more than two per cent, one per cent and 12 per cent globally and two per cent, one per cent and 15 per cent respectively in Asia. Untreated reproductive tract infection, including pelvic inflammatory, diseases, sexually transmitted diseases particularly 'Chlamydia' and 'Trachomitis' and 'Gonorrhoea', and botched or repeated abortions were also known correlates of infertility among women. The results of the multicentric WHO study (1994) suggested that in Asia, among women with a demonstrable cause, almost half have probably become infertile as a result of either sexually transmitted diseases (STD) or unsafe management of abortion or delivery. Among men with a demonstrable cause, about one-third was probably infertile as a result of STD experience. There was considerable variation in a contribution of previous history of STD to infertility. Its contribution had been, therefore considerably lower among infertile couples in Asia than in Africa (13%). In Africa and other countries with high risk factors, two-thirds of infertile women who were never pregnant were reportedly infertile because of previous pelvic infection, mostly sexually transmitted. This compares with roughly one-third in other settings. The most frequent cause of male infertility was inflammatory disease of male accessory glands (12.9%). In 8.6 per cent of cases, infection resulted in obstructive azoospermia. Almost half have probably become infertile as a result of either sexually transmitted disease (STD).

In North India, Singh et al. (1996) studied a total of 129 infertile couples, 60 with primary infertility and 69 with secondary infertility were identified among the total 4,453 eligible couples registered at the Primary Health Centre. It was found that among the 69 secondary infertility cases, 58 per cent had one living child; only one couple had two living children. Ten per cent had lost their children and were issueless. About

27.5 per cent had an abortion history, 7 per cent had stillbirths and 4 per cent had both abortions and stillbirth. It was found that genital tuberculosis was major etiological factor in infertility. Parikh et al. (1997) reviewed 300 infertile women with tubule damage examined at a research centre in Mumbai. The duration of infertility ranged from 5 to 15 years. The underlying causes of tubule infertility in their series were pelvic inflammatory disease other than tuberculosis (106 women or 35%), pelvic tuberculosis (117 women or 39%), endometriosis (63 women or 21%), previous tubule ectopic frequency (8 women or 3%) and previous abdominopelvic surgery (6 women or 2%), 19 women had evidence of simple tubule blockage, 46 (15.3%) showed tubo-overion masses and 72 (23.9%) had a frozen pelvis. Of the 104 women counselled about *in vitro* fertilisation (IVF), 34 under went the procedures; the pregnancy rate was 16.6 per cent per transfer.

PREVALENCE OF INFERTILITY

According to a WHO report (1991), it is estimated that between 8 and 12 per cent of couples experience some form of infertility during their reproductive age, thereby affecting 50 to 80 million people. In a core of about 5 per cent of cases, the causes of infertility are attributed to anatomical, genetic, endocrinological or immunological factors. The remaining 3 to 7 per cent is the consequence of sexually transmitted diseases or of complications suffered post-partum or post-abortion. Studies in developed countries suggest that about 15 per cent of couples experience primary or secondary infertility at some time in their reproductive lives, and about half of these couples do not succeed in bearing (more) children (Jejeebhoy, 1998).

A global review of infertility from World Fertility Survey (WFS) and other sources estimates similar rates of infertility in South Asia (Bangladesh 4%, Nepal 6%, Pakistan 5%, Sri Lanka 4%). Estimates for other regions of the world also fall, by and large between 3 and 6 per cent. Infertility in Middle East, Latin America, and Europe is estimated 3 per cent while it is 5-6 per cent in North America and Caribbean. In contrast, estimates for Africa are higher around 10 per cent (Farely and Balsey, 1998).

In fact, there is little evidence on the levels of patterns of infertility in India and South Asia, more generally, and the little that is available is not necessarily reliable and comes largely from measures of childlessness drawn from census and surveys. The recent National Fertility Health Survey (NFHS), for example, estimates childlessness at 2.4 per cent of currently married women over 40 in India. The 1981 Census of India estimates infertility to be in the range of 4-6 per cent (Vaessen, 1984; Farely and Balsey, 1998).

The prevalence of infertility and its etiological factors in Egypt were studied by The Egyptian Fertility Care Society (EFCS) in 1995. Sample of the study consisted of 768 couples reporting primary infertility. It was found that a large number of infertile men and particularly women sought modern health services for infertility, i.e., 43 per cent of husbands and 73 per cent of wives sought medical treatment; 6 per cent of husbands and 16 per cent of wives also sought care from traditional healers substantiating the reliance on traditional medicine particularly for women. Using methodological approaches recommended by WHO, Phillippoy and Osetal (1998) examined the epidemiology and causes of infertility in Tomble, Western Siberia. The study was based on the findings of a randomly selected sample of 2,000 married women aged 18-45 years. The study was executed in two stages; the first involved selective epidemiological investigation followed by data processing; the second consisted of clinical evaluation of the infertile couples. Among the respondents 333 couples were considered infertile since they had not conceived after 12 months or more of unprotected intercourse. This group of infertile couples was offered comprehensive clinical investigations but only 186 couples completed this. It was found that infertility rate in Tomble was 16.7 per cent, and it was caused by disease of the female reproductive system in 52.7 per cent of the couples and by male reproductive diseases in 6.4 per cent cases. In 38.7 per cent of couples, both spouses suffered from infertility, while in 2.2 per cent case causes of infertility were not determined. Among the cases of female infertility, secondary infertility dominated (12.9% of all the women questioned), while primary tubule potency (36.5%) and pelvic adhesions (23.6%) and endocrine pathology was found in 32.8 per cent of cases. The most frequent cause of male infertility was inflammatory disease of male accessory glands (12.9%). In 8.6 per cent of cases, infection resulted in obstructive azoospermia. Varicocele was registered in 11.3 per cent of cases and idiopathic pathospermia in 20.9 per cent. Inflammatory complications among females were 4.2 times more frequent than among females.

GOALS FOR CHILDBEARING

Parents give number of reasons for having children. These include carrying on the family name, fulfilling the self, expanding the self by giving a purpose to life, providing a learning experience, love, fun and stimulation, conferring adult status on the parents and giving something useful to do, and self-satisfaction of parents. Children provide emotional satisfaction, fun of playing, companionship, happiness and satisfaction to parents along with continuation of family and tradition. The goals, which signify financial addition to the family resources, were classified under economic goals.

In order to find out the goals of having children, Singh et al. (1981) explored the questions of why humans want children by dwelling into biological, cultural, political and economic motivations. It was found that specifically addressed were personal reasons for wanting children, the sense of having a power over another, and the demonstration of competence in an essential role, status and personal leisure. Hoffman and Mani (1979) extended the analysis further covering nine countries and found parents giving number of reasons for having children. These included carrying on the family name, fulfilling the self, expanding the self by giving a purpose to life, providing a learning experience, love, fun and stimulation, conferring adult status on the parents and giving something useful to do. While few parents directly cited the moral worth of being a parent putting the needs of others first and becoming less selfish, 3 per cent of the mothers and 11 per cent of the fathers indicated that they felt parenthood had made them better and less selfish people.

The goals of having children are classified by Sharma (1999) as follows:

Responsibility Goals

Most of the parents valued these goals most fervently. They felt a responsibility towards their lineage and the all powerful creator God. They had to bring forth children to overcome their debt to their ancestors and if they did not bring children into their world, they would be annoying God.

Safety Goals

Safety goals were those that enhance the security of parents and families. It secures their status as parent and the family remains intact if these goals were met. These included identity, security, strengthening, marriage bonds and family ties.

Emotional Goals

Emotional goals were the personal goals of parents related to their own self, fulfilment of parenthood, source of joy, expression of self, and relief from loneliness. These goals of having children were related to emotional satisfaction of parents.

Economic Goals

The goals, which signify financial addition to the family resources, were classified under economic goals. With more hands to earn and economic help, these goals signify children as economic assets.

BELIEFS ABOUT CHILDLESSNESS

There are many popular beliefs associated with childlessness. In different cultures, people have tried to explain the causes of infertility in varied ways. Every land has its set of customs and folklore for the relief of infertility.

In South India, there is a superstition that if a barren woman wears a saree of an expectant mother, soon after the performance of religious ceremony meant for expectant couple, she will definitely conceive. It is believed that if a woman has no child, snake worship will bless her with a child. Women worship the idols installed under the Pipal tree, smear them with sandal paste, turmeric powder and kum-kum, they go around the tree 108 times known, as *Aswatta Pradakshana*. Vedic Brahmins officiate at the ceremony. Once the woman becomes a mother, she instals a snake-stone image under the tree (Ramakrishna, 1989).

Certain deities of the Hindu pantheon are supposed to be susceptible to the prayers of barren women who invoke the desired blessings of fruitfulness. The seven pagodas between Chennai and Masulipattnam are a particularly favoured place for this purpose. On the banks of Ganges, too, at Banaras, close to Nepal temple and burning Ghats, there is a huge recumbent of the figure of god *Bhim,* which is believed to posses peculiar virtues in this direction at a particular season (Kaul, 1996).

A famous deity of Bengali women is Shasthis, the protector of woman, children, and healthy maternity. She may be worshipped with or without image and the worship may be carried out without a priest. Barren women make offerings and prayers to her. Sometimes she is represented by a Banyan stick in a lump of clay to which artificial flowers are offered (Margaret, 1987).

In Gunnu ritual of the Nupe of West Africa, childless women are not allowed to attend the rest of the ritual, and are visited in their huts and lashed as a punishment and as a promise of fertility (Bennett, 1965). In order to improve fertility, Chinese women are given dried placenta to eat to improve their fertility (Donald, 1963).

There are many other measures in different parts of the country which are believed to possess this same efficacy, and to them, in all faith and with much preliminary preparation of fasting and devotion, thousands make yearly journey in the fond hope of being blessed with a child.

RELIGIOUS AND SOCIAL MOTIVES

Procreation is socially desirable for religious and family reasons. Children ensure the continuation of the family lineage. An exploratory study was conducted to examine the socio-psychological mechanisms and motives concerned with desire for children. Five motives were considered, namely, personal, religious, social, economic and health in an interview schedule administered to 50 husbands and their wives. It was found that in case of wives, the religious and social motives played a significant role while for their husbands; personal, economic and social motives were found more important (Dixit and Mathur, 1976). Another study attempted in 1982 to find out why people decide to bring children into the world. To find 'wrong' and 'right' reasons for having children, researchers studied 199 married couples who ranged from having no children to being parents of four. The major motivations of childbearing were the reasons for a close relationship with another human being and to wish to take part in education and training of a child. The major deterrents were the expenses connected with children and parents' perception that a child would interfere with their educational and vocational goals (Campbell et al., 1982).

According to Reddy and Mahadeven (1986), statistical data may explore parental values attached to male and female children. An overwhelming majority considered male-child necessary for old age security (89%), performing death rituals (82%), management of family (79%), maintaining the family lineage (75%). The female children were associated with household work (86%), enjoyment to parents (76%) giving respect to elders (70%) and old age security (72%). Hoffman (1988) attempted an international study of the value of children to parents in the nine countries. Parents were asked to describe the 'good' things about having children compared with not having children at all. The good things most often mentioned were parents' need for economic help, primary ties and affection, stimulation and fun, expression of self and adult status of social identity. The frequencies with which various needs were mentioned however varied considerably from country to country. On the whole, the utilisation value of children was mentioned more often in countries and regions with predominantly rural economies as compared to those with industrialised economies. At the base, the critical quality was probably not rural vs. urban 'per se' so much as the level of income and the availability of other forms of support for parents.

There are also studies to explore the advantages and disadvantages of bearing children. A study of Arnold (1977) covered six countries, namely, Taiwan, China, Japan, Korea, Philippines, Thailand, and Hawaii Islands of US. The advantage of having children were identified as emotional satisfaction, fun of playing with children, companionship, happiness and satisfaction to parents, continuation of family and tradition, providing help to their parents in old age and self-satisfaction of parents. The disadvantages were financial cost of child-rearing, emotional and opportunity costs, the cost on education, noise and disorder caused by children, health problems of children, the problem of physical work and fatigue caused by them, lack of freedom to do as they wished, restrictions on parent's time and career.

MARITAL LIFE OF CHILDLESS COUPLES

Fertility is regarded as a blessing and barrenness as a curse. Barrenness represents a potentially serious source of maladjustment in many couples regardless of their educational attainment, and socio-economic status. When barrenness was involuntary, the husband and the wife tried to blame each other for inability to produce offspring. Some studies show that the status of the childless women depends upon their economic and educational status. Among the poor women with little or no education, the failure to have any children would certainly lead to divorce or a remarriage on the part of husband. Childlessness also leads to polygamous marriages. Some wives, allow their husbands to marry a second wife when it becomes clear that they are barren.

According to Morris (1972), procreation is one of the major aims of marriage among African families. There is an extreme concern among African families to have as many children as they can. Fertility is regarded as a blessing and barrenness as a curse and the Nigerian couples would take all necessary measures including sacrifices before gods, consulting medical professionals, herbalists and divines to ensure that the curse of barrenness is removed. Barrenness represents a potentially serious source of maladjustment in many Nigerian couples regardless of their educational attainment, and socio-economic status. Daniel studied in 1982, the marital adjustment of involuntarily childless women, and women who were mothers in northern Nigeria. The hypothesis tested was that there would be higher marital adjustment among mothers than among involuntarily childless women as measured by Spanier's Dyadic Adjustment scale. Results indicated that the two groups of women differ significantly in their level of marital adjustment. Mothers scored at a significantly higher level of marital adjustment than did involuntarily childless women. Further investigations showed that mothers were more congruent with their spouse regarding value systems, socio-economic status, emotional stability and self-concept. There were more similarities regarding attitudes and personal value systems between mothers and their spouses than involuntarily childless women and their spouses. This study has thus shown that northern Nigerian mothers show a higher level of marital adjustment than involuntarily childless women.

A newly married woman, who enters the household, does so as a subordinate to her mother-in-law and sister-in-law. Her status in this hierarchy will improve only with the birth of a child. Barrenness, on the other hand, brings social disgrace, excludes the women from participation in religious and fertility rites and can often be legitimate grounds for polygamy. Abdullah and Zeidenstein (1982) found that in South Asia, the demand for children is high because they all are means of achieving an elevated status, particularly for woman.

It was also observed that couples with a low standard of living go more often for second marriages as compared to other couples. In Garo tribe, barrenness of a wife prompts the husband to take another wife, as marriage among the tribal people is generally taken as successful only after bearing children. A man may opt for second marriage if the first wife is barren. Many a time, a barren wife herself encourages her husband to keep another wife in order to have children who would carry forward the family or the clan name (Mann, 1996). Even among Toda of Nigerian hills where the women hold a decidedly low position than the men, a mother is considered superior in status as compared with other women. Sharma (1998) observed that motherhood confers a special status to a tribal woman. She is like a fruit-bearing tree. She must be treated with care and respect. As soon as a child is born, the marriage between a man and a woman is considered successful. It proves the versatility of man and fertility of woman. A sterile woman is not looked upon with favour and in such a case man is free to marry again even without divorcing the barren wife.

Unisa (1999) studied the consequences of childlessness for women with special reference to marital instability in Ranga Reddy district of Andhra Pradesh. It was found that 12 per cent of husbands already had more than one wife due to childlessness. The situation was aggravated in 4 per cent of cases by the fact that husbands were said to have relationship with other women, thereby further risking the stability of their marriages. Only 4 per cent of husbands were reported to want a divorce because of childlessness, showing the abandonment or expulsion of wife is not very common; and 16 per cent reported to have talked about taking a second wife. The impact of pressure from in-laws on husbands to contract a second marriage, and negative attitudes among members of the extended family towards childless wives was less significant, as more of these women (60%) were living in nuclear families. It is encouraging to note that majority of women (72%) did not feel that they faced the threat of divorce from their husbands, or demands to agree to second marriages, or the problem of their husbands having relationship with other women. The harmonious relationship among these couples may be the result of awareness that infertility was treated in many cases, and that women alone were not responsible for this condition.

Conjugal harmony is determined by socio-economic background characteristics. Education, standard of living, and quest for allopathic treatment are associated with conjugal harmony. It is observed that couples with a low standard of living go more often for second marriages as compared to other couples. These couples are also less treatment seeking. Educational attainment is positively associated with marital stability of these women. The couples who have better qualification probably have better understanding about the problem of infertility, thereby reducing the unreasonable burden of childlessness from the women. All these factors may have contributed towards building a more harmonious relationship in these couples. It was observed that marriages between relatives are quite common among these women. The main reason for this may have been the reduced burden of dowry according to the parent's desire for better harmony in the marital life of their daughter. But the surprising findings were that marriages between relatives among childless couples were less harmonious as compared to marriages between non-relatives (ibid.).

It is pertinent to point out that infertility may also be a consequence of marriages between close relatives. Thus, marriages between relatives were not favoured though it was generally presumed that woman staying in joint families experience more pressure from their in-laws for remarriage of their son. Women staying in nuclear families had a less harmonious conjugal relationship compared to women living in joint families. This indicates that there is some support from within the joint family, which is responsible for the positive effect. Disharmony of marriages was evident mainly after five years of marital duration, after probably realising that there was some problem with the childbearing capacity of the couple. Thus, counselling around this time may affect the marital stability (ibid.).

The relationship of sex role orientation to marital adjustment and stress among married couples in terms of type of family, type of marriage, years of marriage, employment status of wives and childlessness was studied by Karunanidhi (1994).

SOCIAL STATUS OF CHILDLESS COUPLES

A large number of studies have been conducted to identify the social status of childless couples, especially women. It was found that motherhood was extolled, while barrenness was held as a curse. Sterility spelled social and emotional doom for a woman; she was considered as an ill omen, both for the household and the larger society. It was inauspicious to run into her early in the morning or on auspicious occasions such as rituals of childbirth, wedding and marriage or while setting out of the house to the fields for sowing or to another village or city. These considerations were indicative of her lower status. It was also found that having a child was essential to a woman's health and to ensure her status in her family and village. In giving birth to child, a woman knew she was contributing, as only she could do to the well-being of her family. Cradling a tiny baby in her arms, she felt a deep sense of satisfaction and happiness. Dorane and Wadley (1986) studied the status of childless women of North and Central India, and found childless couples were much pitied and a barren woman was considered as an inauspicious guest at a wedding or a 'Chauk' (infant blessing) ceremony. A married woman with no children was considered incomplete. Fear of childlessness was sometimes so overwhelming that it seemed to become a self-fulfilling prophecy. Childless women go in droves to visit 'Shamans' (magic-spiritual healers) who were believed to have power to bless them with children. Some women felt that a woman's position in her husband's household and in his heart was dependent upon or at least made better by her production of children. A man may seek another wife if his first wife has not given birth to a child.

Neff (1994) explored the relationship between Central Kerala Nair's social constructions of fertility and gender and the Nair institution of matrilineality. It was shown that social responsibility and consequences were implicated in Central Kerala Nair's constructions of infertility, which may be traced matrilineal. Matrilineal kin had the duty of attending to the family god of fertility and to the needs of females of the matrilineal in the interest of fostering progeny and securing the kin group's best interest. Violation of this responsibility, however, might bring powerful negative consequences to all members of lineage. The ritual of *pamintullal* was performed to mollify the gods, while fertility concepts were extended to include other auspicious forms of prosperity. In this ritual, unattached Nair women served as proxy for the well-being of the matrilineal. These unattached women were to the natal kin group symbolic virgins, the life force, which lineage members seek to harness for their well-being. The concept of fertility was thus extended to include marriage proposals, job offer and other health and economic concerns of lineage members.

According to Patel (1994), parenthood confers honour on a couple. One graduates to a status of full-fledged adult only upon acquiring parenthood. Status gradation through motherhood was so marked that barrenness was a dreaded condition. The inferior status accorded to barren women was the other side of a high value accorded to infertility. In quarrels and squabbles, she was insulted for her infertility. The dart of barrenness was thrown at her to whittle down her strength and to latently glorify fertility. She was under constant pressure from household members, relatives and neighbours to produce children. Couples who had children were the most satisfied with family life. The divorced or separated or those having no children at all were found less satisfied. The important predictors of family satisfaction were found to be good relations with friends, with living arrangements and having children.

In most of the cases, women tried various traditional remedies and religious rituals before medical check-up. They believed that infertility was due to the sins of the past life, because they had less awareness of the causes, treatment and alternative in the areas of infertility. Doctors and social workers did not impart any information to the patients. Only women underwent diagnosis and treatment and husbands rarely came to the clinics. Little awareness was found about adoption. Deusoza (1987) studied the psycho-social problems, attitude and misconceptions of people in a south Indian city. Sample of the study consisted of 10 childless women and 10 community members. Result of the study reveals that the women felt a wife's role was to be dutiful to her husband and to bear children. Because of childlessness, women come under severe pressure from her husband, in-laws and the general community.

It was also found that an educated woman was less likely to be humiliated by her husband and in-laws for not bearing a child, because she considered it as a biological defect which could be treated but somewhere from inside, she felt a vacuum, a hollowness which troubled her subconscious mind. Kaul (1996) studied the socio-cultural aspects of childbearing in a society of Rajasthan (Jaipur district). The study revealed that the in-laws often socially and emotionally humiliated respondents two or three years after marriage or their husbands ignored them. Not only humiliation, the domestic violence against childless married women was also reported. It was found that regardless of social class the women were physically beaten by husband and in-laws for the desire of a baby. So, infertility as one of the causes of domestic violence has been reported by Pitter (1996).

A married woman with no children was considered incomplete. Singh et al. (1996) studied infertility in a primary centre of North India. Sample of the study consisted of 129 infertile couples. It was found that more than half of the wives (52%) reported insensitive behaviour targeted to their childlessness from their neighbours or relatives while 35% did not report such behaviour. Fewer husbands (22%) reported such behaviour; the majority (65%) did not, while reporting of this behaviour was significantly greater by the wives as compared to the husbands. The husband reflected maltreatment of the infertile women within the family in the form of the threat of the second marriage. The husbands in two cases refused investigations of self or of the wife. In other two cases, the husbands were living away from the wives while seven of the husbands had married a second time and five of them did not have any issue from the first marriage.

According to Health Ministry of Japan, more and more couples have been seeking sterility treatment and the most common treatment was artificial insemination by the husband.

Despite the fact about one-tenth in Japanese couples was believed to be incapable of producing children, they still come under merciless social pressure to produce offsprings. Getting married and having children were considered what people normally accomplish in Japanese society. Those who were not able or do not want to fulfil this norm become quite vulnerable to social pressure (*Daily Excelsior*, 1998).

AREA OF THE STUDY

This study has been conducted in Rajasthan. The State occupies the first rank in terms of area and the ninth rank in terms of the population. According to 1991 census, the population of the state was 43.88 million. Rajasthan is an area where social status of a woman is valued with her marital status and motherhood. Childlessness is also considered to be a disability, especially in southern Rajasthan, where STs are more in numbers. To conduct this study on them, more stress is given on Udaipur, Banswara and Dungarpur areas. To conduct this study on general category, infertility clinics and doctors were contacted in Ajmer, Bhilwara, Chittorgarh and Udaipur areas. In addition to these, couples visiting private clinics, infertility centres and hospitals in different parts of Rajasthan have also been included.

SAMPLING

In order to draw sample of childless couples, quota and cluster sampling technique was used. The potential subjects were contacted through people like the relatives, friends and neighbours of the researcher. These people who knew about childless couples helped in identifying the sample. Names of childless couples were also obtained from the government hospitals and infertility clinics. Magico-spiritual healers from religious places were also contacted for identification of the sample. Maidservants, grocers were also contacted to identify the sample. All medical specialists in the field of infertility were contacted and only those who were willing to be part of the study were included.

The focus on the socio-demographic and economic profile of the childless couples is primarily based on their age, type of house, type of marriage, occupational status, income, family, etc. Several researches have been conducted taking education as an important parameter. However, educational status is also associated with economic status and occupation of couples.

30 Cluster Sampling Technique recommended by World Health Organisation was used to obtain the requisite information. In the present study, in all 240 childless couples were selected to study the social consequences of childlessness. To explore the differences in social consequences between the responses of sterility samples and infertility samples, they were divided into two categories and 120 couples were chosen who were sterile and rest infertile. Again, this sample was classified on the basis of caste and each cluster included 30 couples, the sample design is given in Table 1.1 below:

Table 1.1
Distribution of Childless Couples

Caste	*Sterile*		*Infertile*		*Total*	
	No.	*Per cent*	*No.*	*Per cent*	*No.*	*Per cent*
General	30	12.50	30	12.50	60	25.00
OBC	30	12.50	30	12.50	60	25.00
ST	30	12.50	30	12.50	60	25.00
SC	30	12.50	30	12.50	60	25.00
Total	120	50.00	120	50.00	240	100.00

DATA COLLECTION AND ANALYSIS

The researcher contacted every respondent personally. For the purpose of this study, the quantitative data was collected first. This was followed by in-depth qualitative data collection, as is the normal pattern in a descriptive study. Considering the nature of the study, household information, characteristics of respondents and environmental factors like type of house, type of family, occupational status, type of marriage that influence the childless couples' behaviour were also studied. Informal discussion were also made to get familiarised with respondents. Interviews were conducted in Hindi. Flexibility of questions was maintained. If the respondents were not able to respond, the same question was asked in a different manner. Interviews were almost conducted in course of informal conversation.

The qualitative methods are by nature participatory and flexible, and can be improvised, if needed. They help in acquiring specific and detailed information on certain issues of significance. This approach has helped in understanding the perception of the family and community regarding childlessness. The qualitative data was collected through case studies and observations. The fieldwork was not done at a stretch. It took more than one year to complete the data collection work.

It was also noted that all the respondents were very cooperative with the researcher, when it was explained to them that the information would be kept strictly confidential. But the issue of childlessness was sensitive and often painful for respondents to explain and relate. The researcher had to win their confidence in order to get relevant information; their experiences were really painful. Some of the respondents totally refused to give information, as they would not be able to control their feelings while narrating their experiences. Only those couples that were found willing to share the information were included in the study.

An exploratory and descriptive sample survey design had been envisaged to identify social and cultural dimensions of sterility and infertility. The stages, as under, were used for this exploratory design:

1. The case study method is a form of qualitative analysis wherein careful and complete observation of an individual or a situation is done; efforts are made to study each and every aspect of the concerning problem (Kothari, 1985).

Case study of childless couples provided qualitative data, which were found very useful. Five case studies were also included in the presentation to represent the qualitative data.

2. An interview schedule was used for in-depth interviews of the childless couples; both wives and husbands were questioned to delineate social and cultural pressures and the outcome of prolonged childlessness.
3. Informal interviews were also recorded. It was done with an objective of finding out the relationship and interaction among the family members and childless couples, and to cross-check the information received from family members and couples through interviews. The observations were carried out in the situation relevant to the study during the process of data collection through other methods. The comments and experiences of childless couples were also included in their own words.

As a first step in analysis of data, research questions were devised on the basis of objectives of the study. The columns and boxes were designed in the schedule in such a way that data entry could be done directly from the schedule after coding. All the filled-in schedules were thoroughly checked before data entry. Data obtained through schedule was coded and tables were developed keeping in mind the objectives of the study where possible. The data analysis was carried out using the Statistical Package for Social Sciences (SPSS, 9.0 version).

SUMMARY

Every human being has an instinctive desire to become a parent and look after the offspring. Being a parent has many rewards and pleasures. For most people, to live without an offspring, even with the loving mate, is unthinkable. Parenthood as a stage of life is characterised by the need to look after, to take care, to give both materially and in terms of affection. For a woman, it is also an expression of creativity and has both biological and psychological roots. It is evident from our holy books, old stories and myths, how people were blessed with children after praying and fasting and performing various types of religious rituals. Fertility or ability to produce children has a positive social value. Procreation is socially desirable for religious and family reasons. Children ensure the continuation of the family lineage.

Many conditions are known to cause or to contribute to childlessness. Contrary to the popular belief that childlessness is due to some physical problem in the woman, when studied scientifically, the causes of childlessness may be found in both men and women. The causes of childlessness can be physical as well as psychological and sexual. Sometimes all other factors are positive and yet conception does not take place. This may be due to circumstantial factors. Such problems are reflected among cases that often seek the help of the counsellor, when on medical investigation all tests give positive results and yet conception does not occur. It is also seen that certain genetic or social factors seem to be correlated with infertility.

The actual definition of infertility is somewhat elastic; the classical period of time is usually taken to be two years after a healthy marriage, without any contraception. But, in well over half the patients attending an infertility clinic for the first time, the period of infertility, is shorter than this. The relative speed with which the investigations are carried out can be slightly flexible, depending upon both, the age of the patient and the duration of the condition. Generally, couples who do not bear children within few years of their marriage start worrying. The lack of uniform definitions has hounded research on childlessness while it is clear that infertility, childlessness or sterility all refer to the inability of a couple to conceive or bear a child when desired. Infertility is failure to conceive and produce a child. It is slightly different from the term 'sterility' which is inability to conceive and produce a child, where, after all the necessary investigation it has been confirmed that conception is not possible.

Sterility and infertility have negative social values in the Indian culture. Formerly, these were viewed as a disgrace and a mark of shame. In many societies, wife often has no status until she becomes a mother. The infertile couples' relatives and friends did not give genuine support in majority of the cases. Pregnant women and other people's children often evoked negative feelings among them. The social consequences of infertility impose serious emotional effect on the infertile couple, especially, the women. There is social and cultural deprivation, and divorce is its major outcome. The individual finds it difficult to interact with spouses, families, friends and acquaintances. The infertile couples generally lie deliberately and reject social exchanges. They do not get genuine support from the relatives and friends and have negative feelings towards pregnant women and other's children.

References

Abdullah, A. and Zeidenstein, D. (1982). *Rites and Ceremonies of Hindus and Muslims.* Amar Prakashan, Delhi.

Abse, D. (1966). Psychiatric Aspects of Human Male Infertility. *American Journal of Fertility and Sterility.*

Adler, J. (1985). Psychological Reactions to Infertility. *Sex Roles and Coping Styles.*

Anand, U. (1984). Infertility and Infertility Counselling. *Journal of Family Welfare.*

Allison, and Janet, R. (1979). Roles and Role Conflict of Women in Infertile Couples. *Psychology of Women Quarterly.*

Arnold, N. (1977). Infant and Environment. *Journal of Comparative Family Studies.*

Baginski, Bodo J. and Shalila Sharamon (1999). *Reiki: Universal Life Energy.* B. Jain Publishers Pvt. Ltd., New Delhi.

Bell, J. (1981). Psychological Problems Among Patients Attending the Infertility Clinic, *Journal of Psychosomatic Research.*

Bennett, F.J. (1965). The Social, Cultural and Emotional Aspects of Sterility in Women in Buganda. *Fertility and Sterility.*

Brand, H.J. (1981). The Influence of Sex Difference of the Acceptance of Infertility. *South African Journal of Psychology.*

Butterworth's Medical Dictionary (1990). Butterworth and Co. (Publishers) Limited, English Language Book Society.

Campbell, F.L., Towner, B.D. and Beach, L.R. (1982). Cited by Diana E. Papila and Salley Wandkos, *Human Development* (3rd Edition). Tata McGraw Hill Publication Inc. Pvt. Ltd., New Delhi.

Churchill's Medical Dictionary (1981). Churchill Livingstone, New York, Edinburgh, London, Melbourne.

Collin's Concise Encyclopaedia (1984). Peerage Books, London.

Danbick, and Judith, C. (1987). Psychological and Relationship Changes of Couples Undergoing the Infertility Investigations: Some Implications for Counsellors. *British Journal of Guidance and Counselling.*

Daniel, Katz, (1972). *Research Methods in Behavioural Sciences.* Oxford University Press, New York.

Daniel, I.D. (1982). Childless and Marital Adjustment in Northern Nigeria. *Journal of Marriage and the Family Adjustment.*

Deusoza, S. (1987). The Problem of Infertility in Women. Unpublished project report. Tata Institute of Social Science (TISS), Bombay.

Dixit and Mathur (1976). Sex Role Preference among Young Children of Rural and Urban Social Groups. *Psychologia.*

Donald, R.H. (1963). The History of Human Infertility. *Fertility and Sterility.*

Dorane, J. and Wadley, S. (1986). Women of North and Central India. *Women in India: Two Perspectives.* Manohar Publications, New Delhi.

Dubey, B.L. (1977). Rorschach Analysis of Impotence Cases and Their Response to Psychotherapy. *Indian Journal of Clinical Psychology.*

Egyptian Fertility Care Society (EFCS), (1995). *Community Based Study of Prevalence of Infertility and its Etiological Factors in Egypt: Three Population Based Study.* Final Report. Egyptian Fertility Care Society, Cairo.

Farley, T.M.M. and Belsey, E.M. (1998). *The Prevalence and Etiology of Infertility.* Paper presented at the African Population Conference sponsored by the IUSSP and the Central Statistical Office. Senegal Dakar.

Galtung, Johan, (1973). *Theory and Methods of Social Research.* George Allen and Unwin Ltd., London.

Gupta, L. and Shrivastava, D. (1982). Infertile Couples and Neuroticism. *Indian Journal of Clinical Psychology.*

Harrison, M. (1964). *A Couples Guide to Cause and Treatments.* Houghton Mifflin Company, Boston.

Hoffman and Mani (1979). The Values of Children in US: A New Approach to the Study of Fertility. *Journal of Marriage and the Family.*

Hoffman, L.W. (1988). Cross Cultural Differences in Child-Rearing Goals. In R.A. Levin, P.M. Miller, and M.M. West (Eds.), *Parental Behaviour in Diverse Societies.* Jossey Bass, San Francisco.

Hubett, N. Blalock, (1970). *An Introduction to Social Research.* Prentice Hall, London.

Jejeebhoy, S. (1998). Infertility in India: Levels Pattern and Consequences: Priorities for Social Service Research. *The Journal of Family Welfare.*

Karunanidhi, S. (1994). Sex Role Orientation in Relation to Marital Adjustment in Stress Among Married Couples. *Journal of Psychological Researches.*

Kaul, S. (1996). *Childbearing: A Social Phenomenon.* Rawat Publications, New Delhi.

Kothari, C.R. (1985). *Research Methodology: Methods and Techniques.* Willey Eastern Ltd., New Delhi.

Lalos, A. et al. (1985). *The Wish To Have a Child: A Pilot Study of the Infertile Couples.* Acta Psychiatrica Scandinavica.

Lawrence, M. (1980). Voluntarily Childlessness, Involuntarily Childlessness and Having Children. A Study of Social Perception. *Family Relations.*

Mann, K. (1996). *Tribal Women on the Threshold of 21st Century.* M.D. Publications, New Delhi.

Margaret, M.U. (1987). *Women of Bengal.* Gian Publishing House, New Delhi.

Martin, E.A. (1987). *Medical Dictionary II.* Oxford University Press, UK.

Masters, W.H. and Johnson, V.E. (1970). *Human Sexual Inadequacy.* Little Brown, Boston.

Mathews, A.N. and Mathews, R. (1986). Beyond the Mechanics of Infertility: Perspective on Social Psychology of Infertility and Voluntary Childlessness. *Family Relations.*

Mathur, Neeta, (1989). *A Psychological Study of Infertile Married Women.* Ph.D. thesis in Psychology, M.L. Sukhadia University, Udaipur.

Mazor, M.D. (1979). Barren Couples. *Psychology Today.*

Miall, C.E. (1986). The Stigma of Involuntarily Childlessness. *Social Problems.*

Miall, C.E. (1994). Community Construct of Involuntary Childlessness: Sympathy, Stigma and Social Support. Canadian Review of Sociology and Anthropology. *Sociology and Anthropology.*

Morris, I. (1972). *The Sociology of Education.* Allen and Unwin Educational Book, London.

Neff, D.I. (1994). The Social Construction of Infertility: The Case of the Matrilineal Nayar in South India. *Social Science and Medicine.*

Parikh, F.R., Naik, N., Nadkarni, S.B., Soonawala, S.B., Kamat, S.A. and Parikh, R.M. (1997). *Fertility and Sterility.*

Patel, T. (1994). *Fertility Behaviour, Population and Society in a Rajasthan Village.* Oxford University Press, Delhi.

Phillippoy and Osetal (1998). Estimation of the Prevalence and Causes of Infertility in Western Societies. *Bulletin of the WHO.*

Pitter, L. (1996). Perception and Attitude of Female Lawyers Regarding Married Women: Section 498A and Related. Unpublished student research. University of Bombay.

Polumbo and Kraft (1980). Psycho-social Dimensions of Infertility. *American Journal of Orthopsychiatry.*

Postan, D.L. (1990). Voluntary Childlessness Among Catholic and Non-Catholic Women: Are the Pattern Converging? *Social Biology.*

Queeny, M.C., Debra, Santon, Ammelic, Sigmon, Sandra, (1997). Efficacy of Emotion Focussed Group Therapies for Women with Fertility Problem: *Journal of Behaviour Medicine.*

Ramachandran, V. (2002). *Socio-Environmental Assessment in Disaster Management: A Study of Public Sector Mining Industries in India.* Ph.D. thesis, M.L. Sukhadia University, Udaipur.

Ramakrishna, N. (1989). Nagapanchmi: Snake Worship to Beget Children. *Social Welfare.*

Reddy, and Mahadevan (1986). Certain Correlates of Conformity. Child Psychitary.

Rosenfeld (1984). The Psycho-social Component of Infertility. *Journal of Fertility and Sterility.*

Shapiro, D.H. and Contance, H. (1982). The Impact of Infertility on the Marital Relationship. *Social Casework.*

Sharma, S.P. (1998). *Tribal Women in India.* Radha Krishna, New Delhi.

Sharma, N. (1999). Nature, Sources and Consequences of Parental Beliefs. Unpublished Ph.D. thesis, P.G. Department of Home Science, University of Jammu, Jammu.

Singh, V., Bhargava, M. and Kumar, K. (1981). The Values of Children. *Indian Psychological Review.*

Singh, A., Daliwal, L.K. and Kaur, A. (1996). Infertility in Primary Health Centre of North India: A Follow-up Study. *Journal of Family and Welfare.*

Slade and Pauline, (1981). Sexual Attitude and Social Role Orientations in Infertile Women. *Psychological Abstracts.*

Unisa, S. (1999). Childlessness in Andhra Pradesh, India: Treatment Seeking and Consequences. Reproductive Health Matters, *Asia Pacific Population Journal*, June 2001.

Upadhyay, Chakrapani, (2001). *Socio Cultural and Demographic Determinants of Reproductive Health. A Study of Tribes of Southern Rajasthan.* Ph.D. thesis, M.L. Sukhadia University, Udaipur.

Vaessan, M. (1984). *Childlessness and Infecundity: Comparative Study,* 31, London World Fertility Survey.

Van Keep and Smith (1975). Involuntary Childlessness. *Journal of Biosocial Sciences.*

White, R.B. and David, (1977). Psychodynamics of Depression: Clinical, Biological and Psychological Perspectives. *Journal of Fertility and Sterility.*

Wilson, L. and Damingo, L.G. (1978). The Social Status of Elderly Women and Men Within the Filipino Family. *Journal of Marriage and Family.*

World Health Organisation (1991), Programme on Maternal and Child Health and Family Planning, Division of Family Health. *Infertility: A Tabulation of Available Data on Prevalence of Primary and Secondary Infertility.* WHO/MCH/91-9, World Health Organisation, Geneva.

World Health Organisation (1991). *Challenges in Reproductive Health Research: Biennial Report.* 1992-1993, World Health Organisation, Geneva.

2

Observations and Case Studies

The present research study is an attempt to explore the social facts related to issue of childlessness. Since childlessness is a problem that affects the couple, the family and the community at large, an effort has been made to look at this issue in a holistic manner. A predominantly qualitative approach has been adopted for study as the major emphasis is on processes involved in dealing with childlessness. A multi-method approach was used for data collection, which involved use of various kinds of methods namely: interview, observation, schedule and case study to elicit detailed and in-depth information.

In order to get detailed information, informal observations were recorded. The observation method is the most commonly used, especially in studies relating to behavioural science (Kothari, 1985). The main advantage of this method is that subjective bias is eliminated, if observation is done accurately. Second, the information obtained under this methods relates to what is currently happening; it is not complicated by either the past behaviour or future intentions or attitudes. Third, this method is independent of respondents' willingness to respond and as such is relatively less demanding of active cooperation on the part of respondents as happens to be the case in the interview or the questionnaire method.

PROFILE OF SAMPLE

The focus on the demographic profile of the childless couples is primarily based on their age, type of residence, house, current age, duration of marriage, caste, type of family, occupational status and type of marriage.

Type of Residence

From the figures shown in Table 2.1, it can be seen that the maximum number of respondents, i.e., 51 per cent belong to the urban set-up. Only 12 per cent couples live in urban slums and 36.7 per cent couples reside in rural areas. It is quite evident from these facts that residents of rural and urban slums conceal their childlessness; and narrow mindedness being the cause, most of them hesitate to take up a medical treatment for the same. They hesitate in giving the correct information as well.

Table 2.1
Type of Residence

Variable	*Number*	*Per cent*
Rural	88	36.70
Slums	29	12.10
Urban	123	51.20
Total	240	100.00

Type of House

The type of house of all respondents is divided into three parts—*kachcha,* semi-*pucca* and *pucca*. Most of the childless couples living in urban areas, reside in *pucca* houses; the percentage is 50.4 per cent whereas, some people living in slums and rural areas construct *pucca* houses, therefore, the percentage of semi-*pucca* house is about 30 per cent. The least number of couples reside in *kachcha* houses generally belong to poor families and due to their poverty they cannot undergo the appropriate treatment for childlessness and this inability continues to be a problem for them.

Table 2.2
Type of House

Variable	*Number*	*Per cent*
Kachcha	48	20.00
Semi-pucca	71	29.60
Pucca	121	50.40
Total	240	100.00

Current Age of Wife

The current/present age of the wife is shown in Table 2.3. Childless women have been divided into five groups which, according to the reproductive age, lie between the age 19 to 40+. The maximum percentage, about one-third of the total sample, i.e., 34.6 per cent, is of the women of the age group 25-29 years. The lowest percentage, about 8 per cent was found in the age group 35-39 years.

Table 2.3
Current Age of Wife

(in yrs.)

Variable	*Number*	*Per cent*
19-24	54	22.50
25-29	83	34.60
30-34	51	21.30
35-39	18	7.50
40+	34	14.20
Total	240	100.00

Husband's Age

Table 2.4 shows the age of all the male respondents. Like women, men's age has also been divided into five age groups. Men below the age of 24 years only 25 per cent, whereas in most of the childless couples, men's age has been reported to lie in the age group 30-34 years. This makes it clear that the realisation of childlessness speeds up after the age of thirty.

Table 2.4
Husband's Age

(in yrs.)

Variable	*Number*	*Per cent*
19-24	6	2.50
25-29	57	23.80
30-34	75	31.30
35-39	57	28.80
40+	45	18.80
Total	240	100.00

Duration of Marriage

This study shows, the tenure of marriage of the childless couples, in tabular form. Couples with a married life of less than three years are very less, merely 2 per cent. The reason for this may be that some couples do not want a child soon after marriage and so use contraceptives or due to certain reasons

Table 2.5
Duration of Marriage

(in yrs.)

Variable	*Number*	*Per cent*
Less than 3	4	1.70
3-8	97	40.40
8-13	68	28.30
13-18	31	12.90
18+	40	16.70
Total	240	100.00

they do not realise their childlessness for about a period of three years. But about 40 per cent respondents with a married life of three to eight years have realised their childlessness.

Respondents, who have had a married life of eight years or more, have also been selected for this study. Couples with a married life of 8-13 years and 18 years are 28.3 per cent and 16.7 per cent respectively.

Caste

According to the research design of the study, the selection of the respondents has been made on the basis of caste. Couples belonging to the general, SC, ST and OBC categories have been selected in equal numbers, i.e., 60 couples each. Also, in every class 30 sterile and 30 infertile respondents have been selected.

Table 2.6

Caste

Variable	*Number*	*Per cent*
General	60	25.00
Scheduled Caste	60	25.00
Scheduled Tribe	60	25.00
OBC	60	25.00
Total	240	100.00

Income

All respondents were divided into four groups on the basis of their family income. The maximum number of couples falls in the income group of Rs 2,000 – 5,000 per month. They are more than half (51.7%). Couples believe that their economic condition has affected their childlessness. Most of them are of the opinion that if they are financially well off, they can use modern means and enhance the possibility to produce a child. Couples earning Rs 5,000 – 8,000 monthly are 17.5 per cent and those earning above Rs 8,000 monthly are 15.8 per cent.

Table 2.7
Income

(in Rs.)

Variable	*Number*	*Per cent*
Less than 2000	36	15.00
2000-5000	124	51.70
5000-8000	42	17.50
8000 +	38	15.80
Total	240	100.00

Nature of Family

Joint family is synonymous to the Indian family, but the study of childless couples living in nuclear families clearly indicates the change in scenario of the Indian society. In the study, 60 per cent couples live in nuclear families and 40 per cent live in joint families. The reasons for living in a nuclear family are: limited place, big family, service and education.

Table 2.8
Nature of Family

Variable	*Number*	*Per cent*
Nuclear	143	59.60
Joint	97	40.40
Total	240	100.00

Husband's Occupational Status

In our society, occupation not only serves as a source of livelihood but also determines the social status of persons concerned. It also determines the behaviour pattern of the individual and provides opportunities for social interaction. When the husbands in childless couples were surveyed for their occupational status, it was found that 45 per cent were service class. There were 33 per cent men who had their own business and 22 per cent respondents belonged to agriculture and labour. It seems that childless couples who are engaged in agricultural field realise this lack very late and also hesitate to go for treatment. Service class males are more concerned about their family health, family size and childbearing time.

Table 2.9
Husband's Occupational Status

Variable	*Number*	*Per cent*
Private business	79	32.90
Service	108	45.00
Agriculture and labour	53	22.10
Total	240	100.00

Wife's Occupational Status

It is quite obvious from the figures, that if childless women were to be divided on the basis of occupational status, the maximum percentage, which is 22.90 per cent, would be that of the service class women. Childlessness in service class women may be due to the constant anxiety or due to induced abortion because of the service resulting in further complications. Apart from this, service class women consult the doctor very often regarding this problem. About 10.4 per cent women have their own business. Approximately 129 women are housewives; their percentage is 53.8 per cent.

Table 2.10
Wife's Occupational Status

Variable	*Number*	*Per cent*
Own business	25	10.40
Service	55	22.90
Agriculture and labour	31	12.90
Housewife	129	53.80
Total	240	100.00

Type of Marriage

To know the marital condition of all the respondents, they been have tested on two bases—homogeneous marriage and inter-caste marriage. But the maximum number of couples, 95 per cent was out of marriage within the caste and merely 5 per cent out of inter-caste marriage. The nature of marriage has been made the second basis. Nearly 13.75 per cent couples among their own caste and inter-caste, are out of love marriage. Whereas couples out of arranged marriage are 86.25 per cent.

Table 2.11
Type of Marriage

Variable	*Number*	*Per cent*
Love marriage	33	13.75
Arrange marriage	207	86.25
Total	240	100.00

FIELD OBSERVATIONS

The striking emotional feelings reported by different respondents were depression, anxiety, irritability, helplessness, anger and jealousy. The emotional responses to childlessness were more intense in those cases where women were diagnosed responsible and where husbands and in-laws were not supportive. One of the female respondents stated:

> Because of childlessness, I feel cut off, left out and feel that nobody cares for me. I feel socially isolated and emotionally disturbed because of the negative attitude of society.

Feelings of guilt were found in those cases where an organic problem was stated as a cause of childlessness. Although the emotional respondents related to childlessness were more frequently visible overtly in case of female respondents but some of the male respondents also reported undergoing extreme tension. However, they did not show it to others because they felt males were not expected to show it off.

Respondent who were diagnosed sterile and those who had faith in God waited every month for some miracle to happen.

During the early years of marriage, some female respondents reported that their husbands were more loving, cooperative and understanding but as the problem was diagnosed, they observed a change in the relationship. One female respondent of rural setting stated:

> I am very much under threat of separation, insecurity, tension and afraid that my husband will leave me or marry again because I am not able to produce a child for him.

Some couples also reported positive interpersonal relations. Their relations did not suffer because of this problem and had become more strong. There was no friction due to childlessness. Instead, their inability to produce a child brought them closer to each other. They had become more caring, affectionate and more understanding had developed between them. There was no threat of strained marital relations. One of the female respondents, whose husband was sympathetic, stated:

> Sometimes I feel very sad about my husband, I keep telling him to remarry as it is all my fault but he never agrees.

In order to see the relationship of childless couples with immediate family, informal discussion were also made and it was found that in those cases where family members were hopeful for conception, the members of the family kept respondents under close watch. They had to face questions ranging from simple queries to sarcastic remarks when conception did not occur. Female respondents reported getting poor treatment and being given a low status in the family as compared to their counterparts having children. They did not get the required cooperation and understanding to deal with the problem from family members and were often made to realise that they were infertile and inferior. Not only family members but the neighbours also kept a close watch over them and enquired frequently about their reproductive status. They also had to face the remarks and comments of their neighbours. Their childlessness was targeted from neighbours also.

CASE STUDY METHOD

To obtain a real and reliable record of personal experiences five case studies were included in this chapter. The case study method is a very popular form of qualitative analysis and involves a careful and complete observation of a social unit, whether that unit be a person, a family, an institution, a cultural group or even the entire community. It is a method of study in-group of even the entire community. It is a method of study in depth rather than breadth. The case study places more emphasis on the full analysis of a limited number of events or conditions and their interrelations. The case study deals with the processes that take place and their interrelationship. Thus, case study is essentially an intensive investigation of the particular unit under consideration (Kothari, 1985). The object of the case study method is to locate the factors that account for the behaviour patterns of the given unit as an integrated totally.

The case study method is a technique by which individual factor whether it be an institution or just an episode is the life of an individual or a group is analysed in its relationship to any other in the group (Odum, 1929). Burgess (1949) has used the words, 'the social microscope' for the case study method.

The case study method is a form of qualitative analysis wherein careful and complete observation of an individual or a situation is done—efforts were made to study each and every aspect of the concerning problem. Names in all the studies have been changed in order to ensure confidentiality.

Case Study One

Rani Gupta got married to Ramesh in 1990. At the time of marriage she was 24 and Ramesh was 28 years old. She was married into an extended family residing in urban area of Banswara. Her husband is the only son and has two younger sisters. The couple was very happy with their married life, as both had understanding and respect for each other. After few months of marriage, the couples decided to have a child, but they were not successful; they waited for few months, but pregnancy could not take place. Rani's mother-in-law suspected that they might be using some family planning measures. She inquired many times from Rani about this and always advised that first pregnancy should not be delayed as it could lead to problem in conceiving later. Enquiries from mother-in-law made Rani worried. As her husband was the only son, everybody at home was crazy about the child. One day mother-in-law decided to take Rani for medical examination; she took her to a gynaecologist. Doctor conducted some tests and after studying the history and results of tests, she disclosed that Rani had blocked fallopian tubes and there were very rare chances of her pregnancy. This was a situation of surprise for both of them; Rani could not believe this as she never expected these results. Her mother-in-law also got very much depressed when she heard about the inability of her daughter-in-law to reproduce, but she did not show negative reactions as she knew that Rani was undergoing through a period of stress and she did not want to hurt her, rather she tried to console Rani and said that they will go out of the State for advance treatment. Ramesh also felt very depressed when he heard about the diagnosis of the problem but controlled his feelings and advised his wife to have patience and faith in God. From inside he was broken, as he never thought in dreams that he would be deprived of the love and affection of his own children. He took his wife to Chandigarh and Delhi for treatment. During the treatment Rani was very anxious and worried as she did not know the results of treatment but Ramesh supported her in every way. He took proper care of her and never made her realise that there is something wrong in her body. After treatment in Chandigarh, doctors said that there were rare chances of pregnancy. One of their relatives in Chandigarh advised them to visit Delhi for treatment. They went to Delhi also, but did not succeed. Apart from medial treatment, Rani's mother-in-law consulted various astrologers. According to them couple had 'yog' (chance) of childbirth but they will get the fruit after a lot of effort, because of the position of the stars. Different astrologers suggested different measures, like one astrologer suggested reading of a particular book daily, one suggested wearing of gems in a ring while another suggested keeping a fast of 'Ekadashi' and do *havana*. The couple and family performed all these measures suggested by different astrologers.

Besides astrologers, various magico-spiritual healers were also consulted. One magico-spiritual healer stated that the family is under the influence of evil spirit. That is why the couple is deprived of childbirth. He suggested a long treatment, which included visiting his spirit centre daily, avoiding non-vegetarian food and also restricted Rani's visit to certain places.

Since the family was religious minded and had faith in God, they visited each and every place which was advised by anybody. They visited some of the places out of Rajasthan but all in vain; they still had hope in God and narrated various incidents where conception took place after long period of time. Although Rani had support from her husband and family, still she had a feeling of incompleteness and felt vacuum in her life; sometimes she felt guilty and blamed herself. She stated:

> I feel very guilty and depressed when I see that whole family is suffering only because of me.

Ramesh also reported that sometimes he felt very depressed and lonely because he loved children very much and when he saw his neighbours and friends enjoying fatherhood, he felt deprived. But he never showed his feelings to his wife and family members, as he did not want to hurt them. Interpersonal relations of the couples were harmonious, they did not observe any negative change in each other because of the problem and they did not have any threat of separation. Bond between them became stronger as the husband was very cooperative and understanding. Whenever the wife was ridiculed of her inefficiency of not bearing a child, he always supported her and consoled her by telling her that it was not her fault. She was not responsible for her ill luck, it was God's wish and if God wants, he will definitely bless her with a baby. Both husband and wife were found to be emotionally stable and well adjusted.

It was reported by Rani and Ramesh that their family members were very nice and cooperative. They never pointed out to the couple that they were deprived of something. Especially the mother-in-law was very caring, as Rani did not face any insult or sarcastic remarks because of the problem of childlessness. Whenever Rani felt lonely or depressed, her mother-in-law came to her and tried to deviate her mind and created positive atmosphere. Rani stated that she had full support from her husband and family and because of their positive approach she was able to cope up with the situation.

Case Study Two

Kanta at the age of 19 years got married to Krishna Lal in 1992. The couple was from scheduled caste, residing in the rural area of Udaipur. They were living in a joint family, having mother-in-law, father-in-law, two married sisters-in-law and four married brothers-in-law. During the initial months after marriage everything was normal; couple had good understanding. Her mother-in-law was strict and she tried to dominate her, but Kanta did not feel bad about it, as she was submissive by nature but real problem started when she took time to conceive. Mother-in-law started inquiring about the pregnancy; even the ladies from neighbourhood and relatives kept a close watch on her. She was inquired by them every month which made her upset and worried. Whenever menstrual period arrived it becomes difficult for her to inform this to her in-laws, because during that period she had to face more psycho-social repercussions. She stated that one day her mother-in-law became so aggressive that she did not talk to her the whole week, then she took her to a spirit centre; there it was disclosed that Kanta had come under the influence of evil spirit before the marriage that is why she was not able to conceive. After this the situation got worsened; now she was directly blamed for childlessness. Her in-laws even started abusing her parents. After few months, her mother-in-law took her to another *Devra* (sprit centre) there it was disclosed that she was barren because there was something in the family of her in-laws and she alone was not responsible. That magico-spiritual healer gave sacred articles to all the family members; he also advised them to burn green cardamom in the morning and evening. Then her mother-in-law consulted an astrologer, who said that there are chances of childbirth but only after 12 years of marriage and advised Kanta to keep fasts. But the mother-in-law was not happy with Kanta and she stated that a lot of money had been spent over her treatment and still there is no surety that she will conceive. Basically she wanted a second marriage of her son, Kanta did not get due respect in the family, and she was ignored and not involved in decision-making. She felt very isolated and lonely as she was less invited at social gatherings and her relations with her husband also got worsened. She had insecurity in her marital relationships, because she observed a change in the nature of her husband. Because of delay in conception, her husband also became short-tempered and started consuming alcohol; he did not take care of his wife and fought over small matters, even sometimes physically abused her. As nobody at home was sympathetic and supportive to her, so she felt very depressed and stated:

> I am loosing my tolerance power and one day I will commit suicide.

She felt very jealous about other pregnant women and considered them lucky and cursed her luck. Sometimes, she thought that she must have done sins in the past birth that is why she was suffering a lot in this birth; she felt more lonely as she was restricted from visiting her parent's home. She considered infertility as a curse and childbirth as a blessing and stated:

> If you give birth to a child you get respect and love from your husband and family, otherwise you have to face a lot of sufferings.

Her best coping mechanism was crying and worshipping God. She stated:

> Whenever I get depressed I cry a lot and after that I feel light.

At the time of this study, Kanta was taking treatment in a famous infertility centre at Udaipur, but she was not very hopeful about her future. Although she had a temporary or curable inability to produce a child, yet she was not very sure that she could become a mother by this treatment.

Case Study Three

Beena got married to Gautam Sahu in 1983. She married in a joint family, having mother-in-law, two younger sisters-in-law and two younger brothers-in-law. After her marriage Beena was very happy because she was welcomed at her in-laws place and everybody was happy about her arrival in the family. She was very beautiful and so the whole family was proud that they had found beautiful daughter-in-law for their family. Initially, everything at the home was normal as Beena performed her duties very well and used to take care of all the family members. Everybody was happy with her behaviour. Since she was the eldest daughter-in-law in the family, everybody was expecting an early childbirth. They always used to talk about children after her marriage. She stated that even after the first day of her marriage her mother-in-law told her:

> We want to become grandparents as early as possible.

Her in-laws and neighbours kept a close watch over her pregnancy. She regularly inquired about any good news and when the reply was in the negative, various suggestions were given to her but when it took time to conceive she got worried; especially the social pressure from in-laws and neighbours made her more tense. One day her mother-in-law took her to a 'Peer' (magico-spiritual healer) for his blessings. The mother-in-law asked him to tell them about the future of Beena. He stated that she would not have the pleasure of childbirth in her life. This made both of them surprised and they could not believe this, as they never expected that this could happen to them. Beena stated that she never thought that she could not bear a child. When her husband came to know about this, he also became very depressed. After few days her mother-in-law again went to a Baba (magico-spiritual healer) and inquired about her. That Baba also stated that Beena had come under the influence of some evil spirit and has very rare chances of her conception. He gave some *Taweez* (sacred articles) to wear and suggested some measures to follow. They performed all the measures with great faith but all in vain. With the passage of time Beena observed a change in the nature of her husband and in-laws. Gradually they became rude to her. She found a difference as after the problem was diagnosed, less importance was given to her and she was ignored. Her in-laws started giving more importance to her husband, and became more sympathetic towards him; she was blamed and abused over small matters. Her husband who never scolded her, not even when provoked by family members, started abusing her. Most of the time he used to stay away from home and remained depressed. Her in-laws blamed her for the condition of their son. She also felt very depressed and isolated. She also felt insecurity in her marital relations and worried that if conception did not take place after some time, her in-laws will arrange a second marriage for their son. She visited various Babas (magico-spiritual healers) to get their blessings. She used to cry a lot, as she knew that the cause of her deteriorating status in the family was childlessness. She was very worried about her future.

After a period of two years, Beena and Gautam consulted an ayurvedic *Vaidya* for their problem. He gave them a medicine made of *jari buti* to eat on every full-moon night. But that was also proved to be a wastage of time and money. On the other hand, family members became extremely impatient for a child. They became very rude to Beena. The couple spent almost Rs 10,000 on the treatment for bearing a child, but till now they are childless. They are planning to adopt a male child of Gautam's relative. The parents of Gautam are not agreeing upon this but the couple says that after sometime everything will be all right. This is the last resort they can adopt to cope with the problem of childlessness.

Case Study Four

Sushma got married to Suresh Sharma in 1995. Couple belonged to urban setting of Bhilwara. Suresh was the youngest son and has three brothers and two sisters. Mother-in-law of Sushma was very old and she wanted to see the face of her grandchild as early as possible; so after the marriage she started insisting for early childbirth. Sushma did not face any problem in adjusting with her in-laws, as everybody was nice to her. After few months of marriage, when Sushma took some time for conception in spite of not using any preventive measures, she got suspicious that there might be something wrong. Inquiries from family members, relatives and neighbours made her more worried.

After six months, Sushma's elder sister-in-law asked her for a medical check-up and took her to a renowned gynaecologist. After certain tests it was found that everything was normal and she did not have any abnormality. After that, she also consulted magico-spiritual healers and tried the measures suggested by them. One day, Sushma's brother-in-law suggested the medical examination of her husband. After examination, the doctor disclosed that husband has some problem that is why conception was not taking place. It was shock for all the family members, especially for the mother-in-law. Suresh also got depressed but Sushma encouraged him. After this, they consulted an astrologer who said the 'SUN' of Suresh was not favourable. Because of his sperm count, which was very high, created problem in conception. He suggested some measures like offering water to the sun every morning, taking bath at holy places, pilgrimages, fasting for three days in a week, etc. Sushma loved children very much, that is why she felt unhappy and lonely especially at functions related to children. At that time she felt that something is missing in her life. Whenever she went out of station, she used to bring toys and she had a cupboard full of toys at her place. Interpersonal relations of the couple did not suffer because of the problem—rather their relationship became stronger. Suresh was very loving and caring and Sushma was also very cooperative. She never made her husband feel that he had some problem, because of which they could not enjoy parenthood.

She even tried to hide the fact of her husband's infertility from others, but in her inner self sometimes she felt very depressed and lonely. In order to avoid this loneliness, the couple tried to make themselves busy with the children of husband's brother. The couple was also planning to adopt a child but they had conflict, as Sushma wanted to adopt the child from her parent's side and Suresh wanted to adopt from his relatives and both of them did not want to adopt a child from an hospital or orphanage. Till the time of writing the book, the couple had not adopted a child.

Case Study Five

Nisha and Mohan belonging to a schedule tribe family entered the wedlock in 1996. They were in love since 1992. Nisha's parents agreed for the marriage only after she completed her studies. Mohan also joined his service as a bank employee in 1996. It was a love marriage but with the agreement of parents. Both the families belonged to the same caste, that is why the parents did not raise too many objections. For two years of their married life they used contraceptives, as they were educated and career-oriented and wanted to enjoy their life for few years. They were also aware of family planning. In 1998, by mutual consent they both agreed to have a child and within two months Nisha conceived. Both the families were extremely happy but after three months Nisha fell ill and the child got aborted. Everyone of the family members was sad but kept consoling Nisha, though Nisha's mother-in-law did comment that she should not have used contraceptives for two years, and the first child should be born soon after the marriage.

After a short period, Nisha conceived again and her doctor advised her to take complete rest. But all efforts were in vain when after two months Nisha had an abortion again. This abortion became a topic of discussion in the family, relatives, friends, neighbours, etc. In the family, Nisha's elder sister-in-law gave her a lot of support; she advised Nisha's mother-in-law and Mohan to go to a renowned Baba; she also took Nisha to a Pandit. The priest asked Nisha and Mohan to bath in Mansi Gangi in the Vrindavan on a no-moon night. Nisha did so and she conceived yet again, but again within three months she had an abortion. At present, Nisha no longer believes in priests or other religious faiths. After undergoing a treatment in Ahmedabad in November, 2000, Nisha and Mohan are living in Dungarpur and are taking treatment from two different doctors. Mohan is still hopeful. They love their neighbour's and relative's children a lot. Nisha has joined a private school so that she may resign when complete rest is required. Nisha is internally shattered by the successive abortion but due to Mohan's faith, trust and hope, she is also hopeful. Nisha's parents have made a wish at many places and have organised many other *pujas* too.

ROLE AND STATUS OF COUPLES

Role and status of childless couples are affected because of childlessness. It makes them feel isolated from family and society, particularly from the friends and relatives who have children. A couple achieves a social status of full-fledged family only upon acquiring parenthood. Status gradation through motherhood is so marked that barrenness is perceived as a dreaded condition. The inferior status accorded to barren women is deeply felt when they are considered inauspicious on auspicious occasions such as rituals of childbirth, wedding and marriage or while setting out of the house to the field for sowing or to another village or city. These considerations are indicative of her lower status. In quarrels and squabbles, she is sometimes insulted for her infertility. According to some of the respondents, giving birth to a child imparts a feeling of completeness, emotional satisfaction and achievement. It also prevents parents from social and emotional harassment. One respondent stated:

> Only after becoming parents, you get social recognition or approval of the society. Otherwise you have to face a number of psycho-social repercussions because of childlessness.

So, children are considered important because they satisfy the parental needs and give them emotional stability and the ability to carry on subsequent generations.

Children are also considered important for strong marital relations, as children help in strengthening the marital ties, otherwise there will be the chances of conflicts, insecurity of separation, remarriage or divorce. Some of the female respondents reported a change in the attitude of their husbands after the problem of infertility or sterility. The change was more in the negative direction; even the harmonious relationship changed into a strained one when delay in pregnancy caused by sterility or infertility was diagnosed. In those cases where the females were diagnosed infertile or they could not produce live birth they had to bear the strained interpersonal relations.

BEHAVIOUR OF FAMILY, NEIGHBOURHOOD, KINSHIP AND COMMUNITY

Family and society looks down upon the couples who are not able to bear children. Insensitive behaviour to their childlessness was targeted by their family members, neighbours, relatives, friends and community. They were under constant social pressure from family and society and some females even had to face the threat of remarriage and divorce. Because of such attitude, the childless couples, especially women, felt isolated from family and society. They expressed the feeling of being excluded from couples having children at family gatherings and other social events. Men also reported the feeling of isolation but women reported greater social isolation, especially when others shared the experience of their pregnancy and childcare in the neighbourhood. The case studies reveal that they had to face the comments, remarks and suggestions of their neighbours and kins. Participation of childless females in social gatherings especially rituals related to pregnancy or childbirth was restricted because these women were considered inauspicious or incomplete. They were called at the time of having food but not invited at the time of performance of rituals. Childless males as such did not report any major restrictions on them for such ceremonies and rituals. It is because perhaps these ceremonies are more female centred and males did not have many roles to perform in these.

TRADITIONAL BELIEFS, NORMS AND VALUES

In many families traditional beliefs, norms and values related to childlessness were still prevailing. In some cases, childlessness is denoted to be the result of *Devta's* wrath because of couples or family member's inability to please them. In the rural setting, evil spirits could lead to couples inability to procreate. Whenever anybody comes under their influences, it could lead to problems of childlessness.

People in urban setting believed that *Karma* of the past birth influences the life of present birth. If someone had performed good deeds in their past lives, then they receive the benefits in future life, but on the other hand, if someone has done bad deeds in their past birth, he would be punished and childlessness could be one form of punishment for bad deeds of the past birth.

RELIGIOUS PRACTICES

Since childlessness was considered as a curse or the punishment of the past deeds of the affected couples and family members so religious measures like praying to God, performing *havanas*, keeping fasts, attending holy discourses, etc., were advised for the affected couples. If childlessness is due to *Devtas* then pleasing *Devta* by various means was also advised. In several cases, couples believed that medical treatment also worked only if one had good luck and if God wanted to give a child to someone. Along with medical treatment couples tried non-medical treatment including consulting astrologers, saints, magico-spiritual healers, visiting various shrines, following religious practices, etc.

SOCIAL AND CULTURAL ASPECTS IN MEDICAL ASSISTANCE

Medical experts stated that females come first for the examination and they were found to be more eager for receiving the treatment. Reasons cited for such behaviour were social pressure on the women to bear children or stronger maternal instinct of women. Respondents reported that they consulted medical experts ranging from simple physicians to infertility experts. Some of them were still continuing the treatment and other respondents discontinued the treatment halfway because they were fed up with the medicines, tests and pain of injections. They considered the treatment fruitless and expensive. In most of the cases, couples had tried various traditional remedies and religious rituals before a medical check-up. They believed that infertility was due to the sins of the past life; they had less awareness of the causes, treatment and alternatives in the areas of childlessness.

Females found it difficult to reveal the medical confirmation of their infertility to their husbands or in-laws, as they were afraid of serious consequences. Male respondents who were diagnosed sterile also reported having the feeling of inadequacy and shame and they found it difficult to talk about their sterility with their wives and others.

Some of the childless couples initiated their treatment with ayurvedic methods and also with homeopathy. These couples did not prefer allopathic treatment initially because they felt that allopathic treatment produced heat in the body and affected ovulation and strength of the sperms. But very soon, after insistence by in-laws, these childless women switched over to allopathic and religious treatments. Rather than following definite sequences of treatment, the majority of couples followed allopathic and religious treatments simultaneously. Some women reported using home remedies. They included eating *ghee*, herbal powders and leaves of *tulsi*.

TENSION MANAGEMENT PRACTICES

To cope with their tensions, childless couples adopted some management processes like withdrawal from people and activities that reminded them of their inability to produce. They stopped attending the social gatherings which reminded them of their childlessness. They also tried to withdraw from the thought of children and tried not to think about childlessness consciously. Many of female respondents who remained depressed and frustrated because of their barrenness stated that they cried many times whenever they thought about their infertility or whenever somebody reminded them or hurt their feelings by passing comments, remarks and taunts. For them crying served as a form of relief.

Many of the males believed that it was God's will that they remained childless as they could not do anything against God's will, so they decided they would suffer in silence.

SUMMARY

The present research study is an attempt to explore the social facts related to issue of childlessness. A predominantly qualitative approach has been adopted for study as the major emphasis is on processes involved in dealing with childlessness. In order to get detailed information and to see the relationship of childless couples with immediate family, informal discussions were also made. It was found that in those cases where family members were hopeful for conception, the members of the family kept respondents under close watch. They had to face questions ranging from simple queries to sarcastic remarks when conception did not occur. Not only family members but the neighbours also kept a close watch over them and enquired frequently about their reproductive status. Their childlessness was targeted by neighbours also.

Although the emotional respondents related to childlessness were more frequently visible overtly in case of female respondents but some of the male respondents also reported undergoing extreme tension. However, they did not show it to others because they felt males were not expected to show it off. Respondents who were diagnosed sterile and those who had faith in God waited every month for some miracle to happen.

During the early years of marriage, some female respondents reported that their husbands were more loving, cooperative and understanding but as the problem was diagnosed, they observed a change in the relationship. Some couples also reported positive interpersonal relations. Their relations did not suffer because of this problem and had become stronger. There was no threat of strained martial relations.

To obtain a real and reliable record of personal experiences five case studies were included in this chapter. The case study deals with the processes that take place in their interrelationship. In order to see the relationship of childless couples with the immediate family informal discussions were also made and it was found that in those cases where family members were hopeful for conception, the members of the family kept respondents under close watch. They had to face questions ranging from simple queries to sarcastic remarks when conception did not occur. Not only family members but the neighbours also kept a close watch over them and enquired frequently about their reproductive status. Their childlessness was targeted by neighbours also.

A couple achieves a social status of full-fledged family only upon acquiring parenthood. Role and status of childless couples are affected because of childlessness. Participation of childless females in social gatherings, especially rituals related to pregnancy or childbirth was restricted because these women were considered inauspicious or incomplete. To cope up with their tensions, childless couples adopted some management processes like withdrawal from people and activities that reminded them of their inability to produce. They stopped attending the social gatherings where they would be reminded of their childlessness.

References

Burgess, E.W. (1949). *Research Methods in Sociology.* New York Philosophical Library, New York.

Cooley, W.W. and Lohnes, Paul (1971). *Multivariate Data Analysis.* John Wiley & Sons, New York.

Kothari, C.R. (1985). *Research Methodology: Methods and Techniques.* Wiley Eastern Ltd., New Delhi.

Odum, H.W. (1929). *An Introduction to Social Research.* Henry Holt and Co., New York.

Young, P.V. (1960). *Scientific Social Surveys and Research.* Prentice Hall, New York.

3

Marital Life and Family Situations

Family is the basic unit of the organisation of human society. If a person wants to understand the formation, administration and working of a social organisation, it is important that he understands family from a sociological point of view. The general or simplified meaning of a family is "a mother, a father and their children who stay at one or different places". In a family, the relationship of a husband and wife is established through marriage. Therefore, it is important for an establishment or construction of a family that a man and a woman, through the recognised institution of marriage and all the rituals therewith, come together and start a family. The structure of a family is based on the relationships of kinship, which are linked together in the patterns of duty and rights, feelings and governance. Emotional thoughts like love, cooperation, childbearing, service are found among the members of the family. In context of the Indian society, joint family is the smallest sociological unit of the social organisation. According to Iravati Karve, if we want to understand the culture of India, it is important that we understand the organisation of three things—lingual area, caste and family. It is true that the nature and the working of joint families have changed. Nature of marriages has also undergone changes—late marriages, love marriages and inter-caste marriages are in vogue. Marriage is no longer a relationship between two families but a relationship between individuals. Youngsters sometimes get married with the cooperation of parents but nowadays, the affirmation and consent of the entire family do not matter much. Similarly, formalism has started creeping into the family life as well. There is a lack of deep and soulful relationship. Love and appreciation have reduced. The new generation does not give much importance to elderly people; they take personal decision and accomplish any big task. The status image of a person has started affecting his family membership.

Many factors are responsible for such a situation, be they the effect of westernisation and urbanisation or the effect of education and the industrial age. But, the family scenario in the society is undergoing a rapid change. Decisions like marriage, childbearing, etc., are now made on the basis of logical reasoning. Consequently, the level of satisfaction of the family has also changed among other decisions for the good of one's nuclear family, the time of having a child, number of children and the gap between each child, are also present. In case of any problem, an attempt is made to solve it by holding discussions between the husband and wife. This condition shows that the role of the family is changing. In this chapter, an attempt has been made to analyse the changing conditions of marital and family life. The level of marital satisfaction of the (childless) couples out of love marriage and their parents differs with that of those couples out of arranged marriage. Sources, concerning the use of contraceptives by men and women for not having a child due to modern education and its relevance in the society, have also been found and analysed.

In the Indian social set-up, having a son is the most important aim of marriage. In the *Manusamhita* and the

Mahabharata, the word *putra* or son means one who saves the father from going to hell. The importance of a son in a family is so much that it is considered as a duty towards the society. So, when a couple gains consciousness towards childlessness, they leave no stone unturned to have a child. They sometimes seek the advice of a doctor and sometimes the help of priests, astrologers, etc., to maintain their religious beliefs. The situation worsens when after conception, the child born is not alive and gets aborted. When the abortion is natural, the couple does not feel guilty. But they are not able to face themselves and feel guilty in their own eyes, when due to some reasons, they deliberately get the child aborted and then in the future, complications arise. The couple undergoes many tortures during childlessness and the hard pressures of parents and curiosity of the society produces dissatisfaction within the couple. The married life and family life of the couple also gets affected due to childlessness and the evident effects are on their relationship. The relationships, which are intimate tend to become boring. In some families, the tension gets so worse that soon struggles develop in the family.

SOCIAL NETWORK OF MARRIAGE AND FAMILY

Marriage in Hindu society, by and large, is considered as a sacred phenomenon. One of the reasons being, that in Hindu way of life, theoretically one complete part of life is devoted to *Kama*, which is both a source of pleasure and progeny. In the case of the latter, birth of son in the family is the most desired thing. This desire is rationalised through the theory of *moksha* (salvation). *Putra prapti* (begetting a son) is essential, as it is the son who is expected to fulfil all the paternal obligations by way of performing last rites and post-death rites (Niranjana, 2000).

As a social institution, Hindu *vivaha* (marriage) is a ritual and a formality, of course, very important, through which an individual has to go, to be able to start his or her life in the *Grihasthasrama*, i.e., the householder's life. The meaning of vivaha refers mainly to the ceremony of 'carrying away' the bride to the house of the bridegroom. Among the Hindus, *vivaha* is generally considered as obligatory for every person; because, in the first place, the birth of a son as said, enables one to obtain *moksha*. "To be mothers, women were created, and to be fathers men; therefore, the *Vedas* ordain that *dharma* must be practised by man together with his wife" (Prabhu, 1963).

The institution of marriage, as per its tradition of marriage, as per its traditionally defined functions establishes a family—the smallest social unit of the society—carries on reproduction, and thereby provides continuity to the society. With its well-defined rules the institution of marriage regulate sexual behaviour of the members. Redcliffe-Brown and Malinowski, by keeping in view such functions argue that marriage and family thus prevent possible chaos in the social relationships. Reproduction, although a biological process, but at the same time is a social and cultural phenomenon also. It is this social and cultural aspect which regulates the sexual life of the couples through a host of social and cultural values (Niranjana, 2000).

The selection of a spouse for a child of the joint family is a matter of deep concern for all the members and usually entails long discussions, protracted parleys, and a considerable expenditure. Certain considerations narrow the range of choice. The prospective mate must be of the same caste as that of the family, for even on the most westernised levels of Indian society, marriages between those of different castes are not common. Usually the match must be made with someone of the same sub-caste. Since within the sub-caste certain families consider themselves to be related, the marriage partner must not come from one of these related families (Stevenson, 1910).

In Indian society the prime social occasion is a wedding, and in the preparation and celebration of this event, members who have strayed from the familial hearth—even whole sections of the family that may have gone off—are usually drawn back into the household for the affair and participate in a common family enterprise once again (Davis, 1942).

The network of friends shapes the relationship between husband and wife and the kinship in which they live. In the major civilisations of the past, it is likely that the kinship network was most important. But though friends may substitute for kin in the modern social network to some extent, certain general relations between husband and wife seem to be caused by the nature of the network itself.

Regarding the mutual relations between the husband and the wife, the *Manu Smriti* has declared that mutual fidelity till death is the summary of the highest 'dharma' for husband and wife. Manu further adds that once they are united by the nuptial ceremony, they must always exert themselves to see that they are never at variance with each other, and that they ever remain faithful to each other. The true goal of marriage lies in "the consciousness of a permanent and unbreakable friendship" (Prabhu, 1963).

From the earliest period of socialisation in most societies, the child is told that eventually he will marry and produce children. Usually, the full privileges of adulthood are not conceded until the individual has produced children. Great effort is expended to inculcate fertility values in everyone. This extensive cultural apparatus, designed to make fertility very much a part of individual's personality needs, is in sharp contrast to the relative lack of cultural emphasis on an individual's taking care of his own life and avoiding death. Death is an intimately personal affair, and apparently human beings need very little special socialisation to try to avoid it. The obligation of producing other persons, to whom we shall owe extensive and burdensome obligations, requires considerable social reinforcement (Goode, 1964).

The religious and moral values that encourage fertility are deeply entrenched in the community and were an important consideration in the couples' decision to procreate. Hinduism values children because of their role in the funeral rites of the deceased parents. Among the Hindus, the predominant belief is that following death, a person's soul can attain salvation and enter heaven only after a son or a grandson performs certain rites (*shraddha*). Failure to perform such rituals is said to allow the soul's recurrent rebirths, thus retarding its movement toward heaven (Niranjana, 2000).

PROBLEMS IN CHILDBEARING

Newly married couples may have put off having children for a few years while they were getting settled in their marriage or their careers. They have heard all about getting pregnant by accident, so they compulsively chose a method of contraception. One day the time seems right to begin their family and they stop using any birth control method. In either case, once the decision is made, they probably smile at each other, count ahead nine months, and imagine taking care of a sweet little baby just a year from now. But the first month the woman menstruates. Another month goes by, and she menstruates again. They both begin to wonder what is wrong. People tell them not to worry. The next month and the month afterward pass and still no pregnancy. Many doctors advise waiting that year before initiating an infertility work-up. Physicians have good reasons for suggesting that they should wait for one year. Some couples simply take six to twelve months to conceive (Harrison, 1964). After some period they find that tension and anxiety are overwhelming. They find that their life is filled with fears about what is wrong. Tension and anxiety are not the only reasons to begin thinking about starting an infertility investigation but there are several other reasons for this. It is found that many couples adopt contraception early in their married life and discover a problem only when they discontinue contraception to have a child (Freedman and Campbell, 1959).

Abortion and miscarriages are other causes of childlessness. For the purpose of minimising the size of the family, some couples practice induced abortions. Although abortion is legal but its practice is not favoured on account of two reasons. One, it amounts to killing of the foetus, and therefore a sin against God. Second, going for abortion implies something wrong with the health of the woman. This is something, which does not command any appreciation in the community. Sometimes it is the guilt of both husband and wife who have taken steps to terminate a pregnancy for which they were not yet prepared.

The other associated factor is miscarriage, which is more of an accidental abortion. 'Miscarriage' is the lay term for what is technically called 'spontaneous, or unintentional abortion' occurring before the end of the seventh or eighth month of pregnancy. This can happen due to various factors including ill health, fail, or any other accidental reasons. Working in the agricultural fields, doing heavy work and other hazards of life sometimes also lead to such a problem during pregnancy period. Another reason cited by a couple of women holds men responsible for this mishap. The problem arises due to lack of precautions in coitus during the pregnancy (Niranjana, 2000).

STERILITY AND INFERTILITY

In most of the studies conducted till date, be it the medical aspects, social or psychological aspects or be it with respect to childlessness, the conclusions have been drawn on the consideration of infertility and sterility as synonymous. Infertility and sterility literally have the same sense, that is, the inability to produce a child. If infertility is the failure to conceive or produce a child, sterility is the inability to conceive and produce a child.

But in the context of the Indian society, if these two terms are viewed from a sociological viewpoint, their definitions clearly bring out their effect. Infertility is that condition in which the woman can still conceive; she is not considered as *Banjh* or dry womb. Her status and situation is not stigmatised in her family, kinship and society. But sterility is barrenness; it is a stigma for her. A woman who can neither give her family an heir nor can bring continuity in the society is a curse, a bane in the eyes of her husband, family and the society as a whole; her life will always be incomplete due to lack of motherhood. Due to her own sterility or her husband's sterility, she is not considered worthy to attend family, religious or social occasions, as her presence in the occasions is considered inauspicious. People even consider looking at her, especially in the morning, as inauspicious. Such a woman is addressed as barren, dry womb or a cursed womb. The other women of the family keep their children away from her. They do not let such a woman come in contact with their children, or their toys and clothes. In fact, this condition shows the actual picture of the childless couple in the family and the society.

In some cultures, childlessness may cast a heavy shadow on the physiological and social adequacy of the female and diminish the social standing of the male partner. Whatever the demographic policy of the government and regardless of the aims proclaimed and/or pursued by the society, the individual family perceives its freedom to procreate as a most basic human right. Most cultures regard children as an extension of self, as bearers and perpetuators of the family name and tradition as well as an expansion of one's hopes, aims and strivings. The inability to procreate is thus always perceived as a denial of basic rights, an injustice and a disappointment, sometimes bordering on grief. Infertility is seldom, if ever, a physically debilitating disease. It may, however, severely affect the couple's psychological harmony, sexual life and social function. Even in those societies which made family planning and birth control their official policy and social vogue, the individual couple desiring a child but unable to conceive one feels demeaned, deprived and bitter. The grief of a woman who has failed to bear a live born child is no less in modern society than it was for our forefathers (Insler, 1981).

In both areas of the world, however, the common victim and target of medical manipulation is women. It is women who bear the burden of their own and their male partners' infertility in the so called First World, and their own and their male partners' fertility in the so called Third World. In the industrialised reproductive centres of the west, men often do not undergo fertility testing, never mind fertility treatment. In the East, men do not bear the burden of dangerous contraceptives, nor are they, for the most part, subjected to sterilisation. In India, where massive male sterilisation was tried in the 1970s, the government vasectomy programme was so unpopular that it helped drive Indira Gandhi out of office and was discontinued under her successor. Additionally, female sterilisation is a much more complicated procedure fraught with major complications (Balasubrahmanyam, 1984).

A couple's response to childlessness can be understood as both a crisis and a mourning process. Many aspects of the marital relationships are affected profoundly by efforts to come to terms with infertility, sexual identity, self-esteem, and communication patterns and future life choices. Many couples use denial as the first method of coping with infertility, which often prevents them from moving forward in the mourning process. Anger directed inward in the form of depression and learned helplessness, or outward through expression of rage and bitterness, can lead to depression or emotional isolation. The expression of anger is mixed with the feelings of intense grief and, commonly, somatic distress and guilt.

LEVEL OF MARITAL SATISFACTION

Table 3.1 shows the study of the level of marital satisfaction of 240 childless couples on the basis of various variables. When the research was carried out, a total of 65 per cent couples were found fully satisfied and one-fourth couples were partially satisfied. On the basis of residence, the conclusion drawn was that 68 per cent or most of the couples living in rural areas are thoroughly satisfied and only 7 per cent are dissatisfied. Almost the same percentage can be found in the urban areas also. But the people living in slums of urban areas are not satisfied. The number of such people is more than a third. The reason for this

Table 3.1

Level of Marital Satisfaction

Percent Distribution of Couples by Selected Background Characteristics

Characteristics	*Satisfied*	*Partially Satisfied*	*Dissatisfied*	*Total Per cent*	*Number*	*x^2 Value/ df and Significance*
Residence						
Rural	68.20	25.00	6.80	100.00	88	
Urban slums	44.80	17.30	37.90	100.00	29	30.938/4**
Urban	67.50	27.60	4.90	100.00	123	
House						
Kachcha	62.50	29.20	8.30	100.00	48	
Semi-pucca	59.20	21.10	19.70	100.00	71	13.053/4**
Pucca	69.40	26.40	4.20	100.00	121	
Current Age						
19-24	61.10	24.10	14.80	100.00	54	
25-29	67.50	30.10	2.40	100.00	83	
30-34	56.90	21.60	21.50	100.00	51	17.940/8*
35-39	72.20	22.20	5.60	100.00	18	
40+	73.50	23.60	2.90	100.00	34	
Duration of Marriage						
<3	50.00	50.00	0.00	100.00	4	
3-8	73.20	16.50	10.30	100.00	97	
8-13	57.40	39.70	2.90	100.00	68	30.840/8**
13-18	45.20	25.80	29.00	100.00	31	
18+	75.00	20.00	5.00	100.00	40	
Caste						
General	83.30	8.30	8.40	100.00	60	
SC	58.30	31.70	10.00	100.00	60	26.176/6**
ST	71.70	16.70	11.60	100.00	60	
OBC	46.70	45.00	8.30	100.00	60	

Contd...

Contd...

Husband's Occupation						
Own business	60.80	30.40	8.80	100.00	79	
Service	71.30	24.10	4.60	100.00	108	12.229/4**
Agriculture	58.50	20.80	20.70	100.00	53	
Type of Marriage						
Love marriage	81.80	18.20	0.00	100.00	33	
Arranged marriage	62.30	26.60	11.10	100.00	207	6.120/2*
Total	65.00	25.40	9.60	100.00	240	

* Chi-square is significant at the 0.05 level.
** Chi-square is significant at the 0.01 level.

dissatisfaction is quite obvious—lack of education, medication, and other daily requirements. Even their basic needs of living are not met and it is but natural for them to be dissatisfied with their married life.

On the basis of houses, semi-*pucca* house dweller couples are the most dissatisfied in terms of their marital life. Every fifth couples is dissatisfied. It is quite clear that such people earlier may have been living in the slums of the city. The age of a man and a woman also affects their marital life. Women who are above the age of 40 are thoroughly satisfied with their married life but the most dissatisfied women fall between the age group of 30-34 years.

When the level of marital satisfaction was observed on the basis of the period of marriage, it was noticed that for the first three years of marriage none of the couples was dissatisfied. As the period of married life began to increase, the level of satisfaction also decreases. Between three to eight years of married life, 73 per cent couples remained satisfied. Between 13 and 18 years only 45 per cent couples remained satisfied. The most important or prominent reason for dissatisfaction is childlessness together with the defiance of the society due to childlessness. Not being able to fulfil the expectations of the family members also perturbs the couples. The dissatisfaction is the highest when a child is not conceived even after 13 years of married life.

Although education awareness, medication and westernisation have made everyone equal in society, yet among scheduled castes and scheduled tribes one out of 10 couples have been found to be dissatisfied. In the general caste category, most of the couples were satisfied. Men running their own business are satisfied in their families. But in families where the men are involved in agriculture, the couples are dissatisfied. One out of every five couples is dissatisfied. The basic cause of this dissatisfaction is the rural background of these families.

Couples out of love marriage do not let childlessness hinder their married life. Thus, more than 80 per cent of such couples are satisfied with their marital life, while the remaining are partially satisfied. Couples out of arranged marriage, only 60 per cent couples are satisfied, may be because the remaining blame this kind of marriage for their childlessness.

Deep association was found between the type of residence and marital satisfaction. Chi-square test was conducted and significance level was found at .01 level. No significant difference was found on the basis of type of family, wife's occupation, age of husband.

PARENTS' SATISFACTION

The information collected from childless couples about the level of their parents' satisfaction has been tested on different variables and presented in Table 3.2. If seen in totality, not much difference has been found in the various levels of satisfaction. Dissatisfied parents were 33 per cent, whereas about 32 per cent of parents are fully satisfied. The parents' satisfaction was found the most in urban slums, i.e., more than half of the parents were satisfied. Even after 13 years of marriage, 48 per cent parents were found to be completely dissatisfied. Among scheduled tribes, 45 per cent parents have been reported to be dissatisfied. But, satisfied parents are mostly of those couples

Table 3.2
Parents' Satisfaction
Percentage Distribution of Couples by Selected Background

Characteristics	*Satisfied*	*Partially Satisfied*	*Dissatisfied*	*Total Per cent*	*Number*	*x^2 Value/ df and Significance*
Residence						
Rural	30.70	27.30	42.00	100.00	88	
Urban slums	17.20	34.50	48.30	100.00	29	12.671/4**
Urban	35.80	40.60	23.60	100.00	123	
House						
Kachcha	14.60	39.60	45.80	100.00	48	
Semi-pucca	25.40	29.50	45.10	100.00	71	20.743/4**
Pucca	42.10	36.40	21.50	100.00	121	
Current Age						
19-24	29.60	29.70	40.70	100.00	54	
25-29	22.90	36.10	41.00	100.00	83	
30-34	27.50	37.20	35.30	100.00	51	19.843/8**
35-39	50.00	27.80	22.20	100.00	18	
40+	47.10	47.10	5.80	100.00	34	
Duration of Marriage						
<3	50.00	50.00	0.00	100.00	4	
3-8	35.10	24.70	40.20	100.00	97	
8-13	16.20	50.00	33.80	100.00	68	32.624/8**
13-18	29.00	22.60	48.40	100.00	31	
18+	50.00	42.50	7.50	100.00	40	
Caste						
General	61.70	21.70	16.60	100.00	60	
SC	16.70	45.00	38.30	100.00	60	37.755/6**
ST	25.00	30.00	45.00	100.00	60	
OBC	23.30	43.30	33.40	100.00	60	
Type of Marriage						
Love marriage	12.10	30.30	57.60	100.00	33	11.603/2**
Arranged marriage	34.80	35.70	29.50	100.00	207	
Total	31.70	35.00	33.30	100.00	240	

* Chi-square is significant at the 0.05 level.
** Chi-square is significant at the 0.01 level.

who live in *pucca* houses. In cities, nearly 41 per cent parents are partially satisfied. The urban environment and the growing formalities in relationships might have become an hindrance for the parents to express their feelings.

Less understanding has been found between women in the age group of 19-24 years and their parents, therefore, about 41 per cent of parents were dissatisfied. But as the age of the woman increases or advances, this ratio decreases. A level of satisfaction has been found between a woman above the age of 40 years and her parents.

None of the parents of the couples who have been married for less than three years are found to be dissatisfied, but nearly 48 per cent parents of the couples who have completed the marital period of 13-18 years are dissatisfied. There are 57.6 per cent parents of couples out of love marriage who were found to be dissatisfied and happen to be twice the number of the parents of couples out of arranged marriage.

Sufficient difference has been found on the basis of caste. About 61 per cent parents of the couples belonging to the general category are satisfied, whereas, 45 per cent parents of the scheduled tribes have been found to be dissatisfied. Therefore, when all these levels of satisfaction were measured through the Chi-square test, it was found that residence, house, age of men and women, caste and nature of marriage affect the level of satisfaction of parents. And the significant difference was found to be at 0.01 level.

VIEWS ABOUT PRODUCING A CHILD

The views about having a child after marriage have been divided into three parts and are shown in Table 3.3. The percentage of couples who wanted to have a child early after marriage is more than half, i.e., 52 per cent, whereas about 14 per cent couples are such who have not decided anything in this regard. When the couples who want a child early were studied, it was found that more than 73 per cent rural couples and 68 per cent couples living in *kachcha* houses take such

Table 3.3
Views About Producing a Child
Percentage Distribution of Couples by Selected Background Characteristics

Characteristics	*Early*	*After Sometime*	*Not Decided*	*Total Per cent*	*Number*	x^2 *Value/df and Significance*
Residence						
Rural	73.90	18.10	8.00	100.00	88	
Urban slums	62.10	24.10	13.80	100.00	29	34.014/4**
Urban	34.10	47.20	18.70	100.00	123	
House						
Kachcha	68.80	14.60	16.60	100.00	48	
Semi-pucca	60.60	23.90	15.50	100.00	71	20.872/4**
Pucca	40.50	47.10	12.40	100.00	121	
Caste						
General	38.30	43.30	18.40	100.00	60	
SC	50.00	36.70	13.30	100.00	60	13.408/6*
ST	55.00	25.00	20.00	100.00	60	
OBC	65.00	30.00	5.00	100.00	60	
Husband's Occupation						
Own business	40.50	45.60	13.90	100.00	79	
Service	44.40	40.70	14.90	100.00	108	35.053/4**
Agriculture	84.90	1.90	13.20	100.00	53	
Wife's Occupation						
Own business	48.00	32.00	20.00	100.00	25	
Service	29.10	60.00	10.90	100.00	55	37.419/6**
Agriculture	90.30	3.20	6.50	100.00	31	
Housewife	53.50	30.20	16.30	100.00	129	
Total	52.00	33.80	14.20	100.00	240	

* Chi-square is significant at the 0.05 level.
** Chi-square is significant at the 0.01 level.

decisions. 65 per cent OBC couples and 55 per cent ST couples want a child early. Seeing the lack of attention towards family planning and the nature of families, the trend of producing a child early can be considered as one of its reason. The men and women involved in farming (about 90%) also want to have a child early and it can be said for sure that they do not believe in contraceptives. Among the couples who want to have a child after some time, 47 per cent were urban dwellers and 43 per cent belonged to the general category. In the couples, where women were found to be working, 60 per cent women wanted to have a child after some time.

Thus, it is clear that the views about producing a child were studied according to the nature of residence, type of house, caste and the occupational status of the man and the woman. The difference was found to be significant at .01 level. The effect of the views on the nature of family and nature of marriage was also studied but no significant difference was found.

DURATION OF CONTRACEPTIVES USED

The respondents were asked about the uses of contraceptives. As shown in Table 3.4, even after all the attempts made by the government and various NGOs to solve the problem of increasing population, 65 per cent couples do not use contraceptives. The information about the period of the use of contraceptives was drawn from the 35 per cent couples who make use of the contraceptives and the given table was constructed. Most of the couples said that only 20 per cent people use them for less than a year, whereas only 3 per cent couples use the contraceptives for two to three years. A very important effect of the residence on the period of the use of contraceptives was observed, whereas, more than 80 per cent do not use contraceptives at all. Only 15 per cent couples used contraceptives for less than a year; lack of education, rules and values of the family encouraged them to do so.

Table 3.4
Duration of Contraceptive Used
Percentage Distribution of Couples by Selected Background Characteristics

Characteristics	*< 1 Yr.*	*1-2 Yr.*	*2-3 Yr.*	*Not Used*	*Total Per cent*	*Number*	*x^2 Value/ df and Significance*
Residence							
Rural	14.80	3.40	0.00	81.80	100.00	88	
Urban slums	20.70	10.30	0.00	69.00	100.00	29	25.683/6**
Urban	22.00	18.70	6.50	52.80	100.00	123	
House							
Kachcha	12.50	4.20	0.00	83.30	100.00	48	
Semi-pucca	18.30	8.50	0.00	73.20	100.00	71	21.232/6**
Pucca	22.30	17.40	6.60	53.70	100.00	121	
Current Age							
19-24	18.50	7.40	0.00	74.10	100.00	54	
25-29	8.40	15.70	4.80	71.10	100.00	83	
30-34	33.30	19.60	2.00	45.10	100.00	51	31.712/12**
35-39	11.10	5.60	0.00	83.30	100.00	18	
40+	29.40	2.90	8.80	58.90	100.00	34	
Caste							
General	25.00	11.70	5.00	58.30	100.00	60	
SC	26.70	18.30	1.70	53.30	100.00	60	17.049/9*
ST	13.30	10.00	0.00	76.70	100.00	60	
OBC	11.70	8.30	6.70	73.30	100.00	60	
Total	19.20	12.10	3.30	65.40	100.00	240	

* Chi-square is significant at the 0.05 level.
** Chi-square is significant at the 0.01 level.

When seen on the basis of caste, three-fourths of the scheduled tribes couples do not use contraceptives and only 13 per cent couples used them for less than a year.

The effect of the age of the woman is evidently seen on the use of contraceptives. Around 83 per cent women, above the age of 35 years do not use contraceptives any more, while 7 per cent women between the age group of 19-24 years use contraceptives for a year or two. In this way, the residence, nature of house, age of the woman and caste have an effect on the thought of using contraceptives, which when tested was found to have significant difference at .01 and .05 level.

SOURCE OF KNOWLEDGE ABOUT CONTRACEPTIVES (MALE)

One-third of the males, who are users of contraceptives after marriage, were asked about the sources of knowledge about contraceptives and measures and the conclusions thus drawn are shown in Table 3.5. About one-fifth of the males got this knowledge from friends. The effect of the time to time information about contraceptives given by doctors was seen on 8.4 per cent men.

In the rural areas, it was usually the friends who were found to be the source of information, whereas, in the urban areas doctors were main source for only 14 per cent men to use contraceptives. The effect of the advice of friends on the basis of caste was evident when out of 34.6 per cent men, one-third of scheduled castes were found to be using contraceptives recommended by friends. The effect of media was found mostly on men living in urban areas and *pucca* houses and on the men belonging to the general category.

Among men who have their own business or service elsewhere also use contraceptives on the information from friends but 12.7 per cent and 9.3 per cent men respectively, gain this knowledge through doctors. On the other hand, among women who are serving (service class women), most of them, about 25 per cent are informed by the doctor and 29 per cent gain information through friends. Therefore, it can be stated that the residence, nature of house and the occupation do effect the source of knowledge about contraceptives. On the basis of chi-square test conducted, significant difference was found to be at .01 level.

Table 3.5
Source of Knowledge About Contraceptives (Male)
Percentage Distribution of Couples by Selected Background Characteristics

Characteristics	*Doctor*	*Friends*	*Media*	*Relatives*	*Not Used*	*Total Per cent*	*Number*	*x^2 Value/ df and Significance*
Residence								
Rural	2.30	15.90	0.00	0.00	81.80	100	88	
Urban slums	3.40	27.60	0.00	0.00	69.00	100	29	30.045/8**
Urban	13.80	22.80	8.90	1.60	52.90	100	123	
House								
Kachcha	4.20	12.50	0.00	0.00	83.30	100	48	
Semi-pucca	2.80	23.90	0.00	0.00	73.30	100	71	27.457/8**
Pucca	13.20	22.30	9.10	1.70	53.70	100	121	
Caste								
General	8.30	23.30	10.00	0.00	58.40	100	60	
SC	13.40	33.30	0.00	0.00	53.30	100	60	29.328/12**
ST	8.30	13.30	1.70	0.00	76.70	100	60	
OBC	3.30	13.30	6.70	3.30	73.40	100	60	
Husband's Occupation								
Own business	12.70	26.60	2.50	0.00	58.20	100	79	
Service	9.30	25.00	8.30	1.90	55.50	100	108	34.691/8**
Agriculture	0.00	3.80	0.00	0.00	96.20	100	53	
Wife's Occupation								
Own business	4.00	12.00	8.00	8.00	68.00	100	25	
Service	25.50	29.10	9.10	0.00	36.30	100	55	67.752/12**
Agriculture	0.00	3.20	0.00	0.00	96.80	100	31	
Housewife	3.90	23.30	3.10	0.00	69.70	100	129	
Total	8.30	20.80	4.60	0.80	65.50	100	240	

* Chi-square is significant at the 0.05 level.
** Chi-square is significant at the 0.01 level.

SOURCE OF KNOWLEDGE ABOUT CONTRACEPTIVES (FEMALE)

A considerable difference was found between the men and women who used contraceptives after marriage and about the source of knowledge about contraceptives (Table 3.6). The hesitant nature and exposure of women may be some of the

Table 3.6

Source of Knowledge About Contraceptives (Female)
Percentage Distribution of Couples by Selected Background Characteristics

Characteristics	Doctor	Friends	Family	Media	Relatives	Not Used	Total Per cent	Number	x^2 Value/ df and Significance
Residence									
Rural	2.30	6.80	4.60	4.50	0.00	81.8	100	88	
Urban slums	0.00	0.00	20.70	10.30	0.00	69.00	100	29	36.653/10**
Urban	2.30	14.40	5.40	22.00	2.30	53.60	100	123	
House									
Kachcha	4.10	0.00	6.30	6.30	0.00	83.30	100	48	
Semi-pucca	0.00	9.90	11.30	5.60	0.00	73.20	100	71	31.872/10**
Pucca	2.50	14.00	5.00	22.30	2.50	53.70	100	121	
Caste									
General	0.00	18.30	0.00	23.40	0.00	58.30	100	60	
SC	1.70	8.30	20.00	16.70	0.00	53.30	100	60	50.813/15**
ST	3.30	13.30	3.30	1.70	1.70	76.70	100	60	
OBC	3.30	0.00	5.00	15.00	3.30	73.40	100	60	
Husband's Occupation									
Own business	2.50	8.90	5.10	25.30	0.00	58.20	100	79	
Service	2.80	15.70	10.20	13.00	2.80	55.50	100	108	41.272/10**
Agriculture	0.00	0.00	3.80	0.00	0.00	96.20	100	53	
Wife's Occupation									
Own business	0.00	0.00	12.00	12.00	8.00	68.00	100	25	
Service	3.60	20.00	7.30	32.70	0.00	36.40	100	55	56.397/15**
Agriculture	0.00	0.00	3.20	0.00	0.00	96.80	100	31	
Housewife	2.30	10.10	7.00	10.10	0.80	69.70	100	129	
Total	2.10	10.00	7.10	14.20	1.30	65.30	100	240	

* Chi-square is significant at the 0.05 level.
** Chi-square is significant at the 0.01 level.

reason for this vast difference. About 14 per cent women learned about contraceptives through media (mostly newspapers, magazines TV and radio). Out of the 35 per cent women who use contraceptives, 10 per cent women got information of the use of contraceptives through their friends. Among these women who are told about contraceptives by their friends, most women are urban (14.4%), women living in *pucca* houses (14%), women belonging to general category (18.3%) and service class women (20%) were known.

When the effect of media was observed on these women, it was noticed that media gives a lot of information about contraceptives to the women living in *pucca* houses in urban areas and this information is used by around 23.4 per cent of women belonging to the general category. The percentage of knowledge about contraceptives through doctors and relatives is very less, which is 2.1 per cent and 1.2 respectively. Among business women, 12 per cent women get this knowledge from family members and 12 per cent women from the media. In total, the knowledge of the use of contraceptives depend on residence, house, business, caste and after testing them through chi-square test, significant different has been found at .01 level.

REACTIONS AFTER KNOWING ABOUT STERILITY

Table 3.7 shows the reactions of the 120 sterile couples when they come to know that the reason for their childlessness is sterility of either of them. These reactions have been tested on various variables and the following conclusions have been drawn. 45 per cent couples hold mutual discussions. Out of all childless couples, 50 per cent couples seek the physician's advice. The percentage of those couples who discuss their sterility in the family is not less; about 33 per cent couples discuss their problem at home. Only 27.5 per cent couples seek the help and advice of close friends or relatives. Similarly, 26.7 per cent couples give consideration to and seek the advice of priests or astrologers.

Table 3.7

Reactions After Knowing About Sterility
Percentage Distribution of Couples by Selected Background Characteristics

Characteristics	*Mutual Discu-ssion*	*Discuss-ion with close Friends*	*Discuss-ion in Family*	*Discuss-ion with Relatives*	*Physician's Advice*	*Counse-llor's Advice*	*Consult Priests*
Residence			**			**	*
Rural	48.90	22.70	45.50	17.00	75.70	0.00	34.10
Urban slums	41.40	31.00	31.00	17.20	81.40	0.00	35.50
Urban	43.10	30.10	24.40	19.50	88.00	8.90	19.50
Current Age	**		*		**		**
19-24	37.00	22.20	38.90	16.70	38.90	0.00	25.90
25-29	39.80	26.50	38.90	18.10	44.60	6.00	21.70
30-34	58.80	31.40	33.30	21.60	60.80	9.80	27.50
35-39	66.70	33.30	22.20	22.20	72.20	0.00	38.90
40+	38.20	29.40	38.20	14.70	52.90	2.90	32.40
Husband's Age	**		**	**	**	*	*
19-24	100.00	50.00	100.00	0.00	100.00	0.00	16.70
25-29	24.60	17.50	21.10	12.30	24.60	0.00	12.30
30-34	49.30	32.00	32.00	17.30	50.70	4.00	30.70
35-39	56.10	28.10	38.60	33.30	66.70	12.30	36.80
40-44	42.20	28.90	33.30	11.10	53.30	2.20	26.70
Husband's Occupation	**	**	**		**		
Own business	64.60	36.70	45.60	20.30	64.60	5.10	26.60
Service	39.80	27.80	24.10	14.80	45.40	6.50	25.00
Agriculture	26.40	13.20	32.10	22.60	37.70	0.00	30.20
Total	45.00	27.50	32.90	18.30	50.00	4.60	26.70

* Chi-square is significant at the 0.05 level.
** Chi-square is significant at the 0.01 level.
Note: n = 120; only 'yes' responses in each category.

When the reactions were studied on the basis of the residences, it was observed that about 40-50 per cent couples, be it in rural or urban life, obviously discuss it among them. The percentage grows more towards the rural areas. In urban areas, the couples discuss it with their friends as well. There have been widespread distances among family members also. Thus, the practice of sharing one's sorrows or mental tensions with their family members has greatly reduced. Less than 20 per cent couples share their troubles with their relatives. A majority of couples consult the physicians. The Indian society is basically centred on the principles of *Dharma* and *Karma* that further leads to various religious beliefs in any adverse circumstances. Therefore, a third of the population (couples) living in rural areas take the help of priests, fortune tellers etc. Although the people dwelling in urban areas view things with a scientific point of view, yet superstition is not completely eradicated. Therefore, one out of every five couples seeks to solve this problem with the help of rituals.

The age of men and women also affect the nature of their reaction. Men between the age group of 19-24 years discuss among themselves. 50 per cent of them discuss with their close friends and also with their family friends. They also consult their physician.

Only 25 per cent of them consult fortune tellers or priests, etc. As the age advances, the percentage also changes. Only 50 per cent couples between the age group of 30-44 years discuss their problem among themselves.

When the economic status of men and women was taken into consideration, the data shows that less than a third of the couples in agricultural occupation discuss between themselves but do discuss it with their family members. Type of house, period of marriage, caste, nature of family, etc., were also the basis of studying the reactions of the couples, but no significant difference could be traced.

REACTIONS AFTER KNOWING ABOUT INFERTILITY

Table 3.8 has been constructed to study the behaviour of 120 couples who desperately want a child but face abortion again and again. The behaviour of couples is affected by many situations where, the significance difference has been noticed. Almost 50 per cent of the total infertile couples hold discussions with each other to solve this problem. They also consult the doctor. Direct relation between the age of women and the behaviour was observed. About 61 per cent women between the age group of 19 to 24 years were found to hold discussions whereas, the percentage of discussion is reduced if the age of women is between 35 to 39 years where it comes down to 28 per cent. Men in the age group of 25 to 29 years are one-third in number who first discuss this problem with their wives. The percentage of discussion with friends is the most in urban slums, the reason being close residence and intimate relationship. Most women in the age group of 25 to 29 years, around 47 per cent discuss their problem in the family but only 6 per cent women above the age of 35 years involve their family members in their problem.

A close relationship was found between the tenure of marriage and behaviour. Couples with a married life of less than three years do not discuss their problem with their friends, whereas those having a married life of three to eight years discuss among themselves and trust their friends and share the problem with them also. The percentage of discussion with relatives comparatively has been lesser on every base; but among those who have had a married life of less than three years, 50 per cent of them have been observed to hold discussion with relatives also. When asked about advice from psychologists or counsellors, it was found that 3.3 per cent couples belonging to general category and 6.7 per cent couples belonging to scheduled caste category go to psychologists for counselling.

Table 3.8

Action Taken After Knowing About Infertility
Percentage Distribution of Couples by Selected Background Characteristics

Characteristics	*Mutual Discussion*	*Discussion with close Friends*	*Discussion in Family*	*Discussion with Relatives*	*Physician's Advice*	*Counsellor's Advice*	*Consult Priests*
Residence				**			
Rural	44.30	18.20	31.80	8.00	44.30	0.00	25.00
Urban slums	58.60	31.00	44.80	20.70	58.60	6.90	17.20
Urban	52.00	27.60	39.00	23.60	50.40	3.30	23.60
Current Age	*	**	**				
19-24	61.10	31.50	40.70	20.40	61.10	1.90	24.10
25-29	55.40	33.70	47.00	18.10	53.00	3.60	30.10
30-34	39.20	17.60	27.50	11.80	39.20	3.90	13.70
35-39	27.80	5.60	5.60	5.60	27.80	0.00	11.10
40+	47.10	11.80	38.20	26.50	47.10	0.00	26.50
Duration of Marriage		*					
<3	50.00	0.00	50.00	50.00	50.00	0.00	50.00
3-8	54.60	32.00	35.10	12.40	54.60	2.10	21.60
8-13	39.70	27.90	39.70	20.60	36.80	2.90	25.00
13-18	58.10	12.90	41.90	12.90	58.10	6.50	16.10
18+	50.00	12.50	32.50	25.00	50.00	0.00	27.50
Husband's Occupation	**	**			**		**
Own business	35.40	12.70	26.60	21.50	34.20	2.50	12.70
Service	54.60	32.40	40.70	18.50	53.70	3.70	25.90
Agriculture	62.30	26.40	45.30	9.40	62.30	0.00	34.00
Wife's Occupation	*	*	*		*		**
Own business	60.00	44.00	48.00	28.00	56.00	8.00	8.00
Service	32.70	20.00	21.80	12.70	32.70	1.80	7.30
Agriculture	48.40	12.90	29.00	16.10	48.40	0.00	19.40
Housewife	55.80	25.60	43.40	17.80	55.00	2.30	34.10
Type of Marriage		*					**
Love marriage	51.50	39.40	27.30	21.20	51.50	9.10	30.30
Arranged marriage	49.80	22.20	38.60	16.90	48.80	1.40	22.20
Total	50.00	24.60	37.10	17.50	50.00	2.50	23.30

* Chi-square is significant at the 0.05 level.
** Chi-square is significant at the 0.01 level.
Note: n = 120; only 'Yes' response in each category.

Even with modern medical treatments, trust in priests and sages has not been vanished. To show this, respondents were asked to give responses and it was discovered that not only rural but 24 per cent urban couples also believe on *karma* and the fruits thereof and are always prepared to perform all the rites and rituals pertaining to this belief. Around 50 per cent couples who have completed less than three years of married life hold such religious faith. This percentage is highest in scheduled castes and scheduled tribes.

The occupational status of men and women affects their behaviours also. About 45 per cent men engaged in the agricultural field discuss their problem with the family members. And 60 per cent women who have their own business discuss it with their husbands while 48 per cent discuss with their family members. Couples who have a love marriage hesitate to discuss this problem with their family members. And 39 per cent couples discuss this problem with their friends. It was also noticed that 30 per cent couples seek religious support. On the basis of the nature of marriage, the occupational status of men and women and residence, the behaviours were put under chi-square test and significant difference was found at .01 and .05 level. But no significant difference was found on the basis of the type of house, caste and the nature of family.

EFFECT OF BACKGROUND CHARACTERISTICS ON ASPECTS OF MARITAL LIFE AND FAMILY SITUATIONS

Marital life and family situations of childless couples are shown in the Table 3.9. Couples residing in rural area and in *kachcha* houses have more marital satisfaction, whereas the mutual relationship of husband and wife is not found cordial in urban slums. Parents of couples residing in urban area were found more satisfied than rural or urban slums. As the age of female increases, the level of marital satisfaction and parental satisfaction also increased. Marital satisfaction was found on higher side between the husband and wife married for less than eight years. But parents' level of satisfaction was decreasing.

Table 3.9

Effect of Background Characteristics on Aspects of Marital Life and Family Situations

Percentage Distribution of Couples by Selected Background Characteristics

Characteristics	*Marital Satisfaction*	*Parents' Satisfaction*	*Early Child Desire*	*Contraceptives Used*	*Doctor Source of Knowledge (Male)*	*Doctor Source of Knowledge (Female)*	*Mutual Discussion about Sterility*	*Mutual Discussion about Infertility*	*Number*
Residence	**	**	**	**	**	**			
Rural	68.20	30.70	73.90	18.20	2.30	2.30	48.90	44.30	88
Urban slums	44.80	17.20	62.10	31.00	3.40	0.00	41.40	58.60	29
Urban	67.50	35.80	34.10	47.20	13.80	2.30	43.10	52.00	123
House	*	**	**	**		**			
Kachcha	62.50	14.60	68.80	16.70	4.20	4.10	39.60	50.00	48
Semi-pucca	59.20	25.40	60.60	26.80	2.80	0.00	45.10	50.70	71
Pucca	69.40	42.10	40.50	46.30	13.20	2.50	47.10	49.60	121
Current Age	**	**	*	**			**	*	
19-24	61.10	29.60	61.10	25.90	1.90	1.90	37.00	61.10	54
25-29	37.50	22.90	59.00	28.90	7.20	0.00	39.80	55.40	83
30-34	56.90	27.50	43.10	54.90	21.60	5.90	58.80	39.20	51
35-39	72.20	50.00	55.60	16.70	0.00	0.00	66.70	27.80	18
40+	73.50	47.10	33.30	41.20	6.70	0.00	38.20	47.10	34
Husband's Age	**						**	**	
19-24	66.70	50.00	33.30	33.40	16.70	16.70	100.00	74.70	6
25-29	68.40	35.10	70.20	21.00	1.80	0.00	24.60	75.40	57
30-34	62.70	13.30	50.70	37.30	10.70	0.00	49.30	49.30	75
35-39	56.10	33.30	45.60	45.70	14.00	5.30	56.10	33.30	57
40+	75.60	48.90	71.40	46.70	0.00	0.00	42.20	46.70	14
Duration of Marriage	**	**							
<3	50.00	50.00	50.00	0.00	0.00	0.00	50.00	50.00	4
3-8	73.20	35.10	49.50	40.20	10.30	3.10	44.30	54.60	97
8-13	57.40	16.20	61.80	28.00	10.30	0.00	52.90	39.70	68

Contd...

Contd...

13-18	45.20	29.00	58.10	32.30	3.20	3.20	38.70	58.10	31
18+	75.00	50.00	37.50	37.50	5.00	2.50	37.50	50.00	40
Caste	**	**	*	*	*	**			
General	83.30	61.70	38.30	41.70	8.30	0.00	43.30	50.00	60
SC	58.30	16.70	50.00	46.70	13.40	1.70	43.30	48.30	60
ST	71.70	25.00	55.00	23.30	8.30	3.30	44.70	48.80	60
OBC	46.70	23.30	65.00	26.70	3.30	3.30	46.70	43.70	60
Family									
Nuclear	66.40	28.00	51.00	35.70	9.80	1.40	45.50	48.30	143
Joint	62.90	35.10	53.60	33.00	6.20	3.10	44.30	52.60	97
Husband's Occupation	*		**	**	**	**	**	**	
Own business	60.80	29.10	40.50	41.80	12.70	2.50	64.60	35.40	79
Service	71.30	35.20	44.40	44.50	9.30	2.80	39.80	54.60	108
Agriculture	58.50	24.50	84.90	3.80	0.00	0.00	26.40	62.30	53
Wife's Occupation	*		**	**	**	**	**	*	
Own business	80.00	24.00	48.00	32.00	4.00	0.00	32.00	60.00	25
Service	65.50	25.50	29.10	53.40	25.50	3.60	63.60	32.70	55
Agriculture	67.70	41.90	90.30	3.20	0.00	0.00	38.70	48.40	31
Housewife	61.20	31.80	53.50	30.30	3.90	2.30	41.10	55.80	129
Monthly Income		**		**	**	**		*	
<2000	62.50	20.80	75.00	13.90	4.20	2.80	37.50	55.60	36
2000-5000	61.50	24.60	41.80	41.10	7.40	0.00	49.20	50.00	124
5000-8000	95.20	66.70	61.90	38.10	4.80	4.80	33.30	61.90	42
8000-11000	100.00	80.00	0.00	80.00	80.00	0.00	60.00	40.00	10
11000+	55.00	55.00	35.00	75.00	15.00	10.00	55.00	20.00	28
Type of Marriage		**							
Love marriage	81.80	12.10	51.50	36.40	9.10	3.00	48.50	51.50	33
Arranged marriage	62.30	34.80	52.20	34.30	8.20	1.90	44.40	49.80	207
Total									240

* Chi-square is significant at the 0.05 level.
** Chi-square is significant at the 0.01 level.

In general category, more marital satisfaction was found. No significant difference was seen on the basis of type of family, husband's occupation and wife's occupational status. Parents were less satisfied in love than those of childless couples, but marital satisfaction level was very high in those couples.

Couples residing in rural areas desired early child and they did not use contraceptive as much as urban residing couples. No significant difference was found in desire of early child on the basis of husband or wife's age. Couples from general and ST category used more contraceptives, as they did not want early child.

Couples engaged in farming wanted more hands to help them so they did not use any contraceptive. But where both the husband and wife were in service, they wanted to plan their family and used contraceptives. More than 80 per cent couples earning Rs 8,000 to 11,000 per month, used contraceptives, as they were aware of their family demands. Male respondents from urban settings reported that doctor was the main source of knowledge about contraceptives. Females of urban slums did not get any knowledge from doctors. Besides this, couples residing in *kachcha* houses were also not in touch with doctors, so they did not have the knowledge on contraceptives. Neither husbands engaged in agriculture nor their wives got any information from doctors about contraceptives.

The couples who were in service got knowledge about contraceptives from doctors. Awareness of contraceptives was found deeply associated with income. Most of the female respondents who got knowledge about contraceptives from doctors were from higher income group. When evaluated caste-wise, males of SC category were more aware about contraceptives than their females.

Because sterility and infertility both terms have their own definitions, their meanings, impact and associations were entirely different. That is why relations and situations have been also reflected in a different manner. Couples residing in urban slums discuss with each other about infertility but not much about sterility. As female's age increases, the discussion about sterility increases and discussion about infertility reduces.

The couples married for more than 18 years hardly discuss about their sterility. An interesting point was found that the husbands engaged in farming did not discuss with their wives about sterility but they in a large number discuss about infertility. On the other hand, wives engaged in service hardly discuss with their husbands about infertility but more than 60 per cent discuss sterility.

SUMMARY

In the context of the Indian society, if these two terms are viewed from a sociological viewpoint, their definitions clearly bring out their effect. Infertility is that condition in which the woman can at least conceive; she is not considered as *Banjh* or 'dry womb'. Her status and situation is not stigmatised in her family, kinship and society. But sterility is barrenness, it is a stigma for her. A woman who can neither give her family an heir nor can bring continuity in the society is a curse, a bane in the eyes of her husband, family and the society as a whole; her life will always be incomplete due to lack of motherhood. Due to her own sterility or her husband's sterility, she is not considered worthy to attend family, religious or social occasions, as her presence is considered inauspicious. People even consider looking at her, especially in the morning, as inauspicious. Such a woman is addressed as barren, dry womb or a cursed womb. The other women of the family keep their children away from her. They do not let such a woman come in contact with their children, or their toys and clothes. In fact, this condition shows the actual picture of the childless couples in the family and the society.

A couple's response to childlessness can be understood as both a crisis and a mourning process. Many aspects of the marital relationships are affected profoundly by efforts to come to terms with infertility, sexual identity, self-esteem, and communication patterns and future life choices. The duration of marriage also affects their marital life. It was noticed that for the first three years of marriage none of the couples was dissatisfied. As the period of married life began to increase, the level of satisfaction started decreasing. When all the respondents were asked about the uses of contraceptives, it was found that even after all the attempts made by the government and various NGOs to solve the problem of the increasing population, more than 50 per cent of couples did not used contraceptives.

The reactions of the couples, when they come to know that the reason for their childlessness is sterility in either of them were also observed. In urban areas, since there is open-mindedness, the couples discuss it with their friends as well. The practice of sharing one's sorrows or mental tensions with their family members has greatly reduced.

More marital satisfaction was found in couples residing in urban settings and in *pucca* houses. After the age of 40, marital satisfaction and parent's satisfaction level increased. Doctors benefited very few couples, as the doctor was the source of knowledge about contraceptives. Couples discussed more about infertility than sterility.

References

Davis, Kingsley (1942). *Changing Modes of Marriage: Contemporary Family Types.* D.C. Heath and Company, Boston.

Freedman, and Whelpton Campbell (1959). *Family Planning: Sterility and Population Growth.* McGraw Hill Book Company Inc.

Goode, W.J. (1964). *The Family.* Prentice Hall of India (Pvt.) Ltd., New Delhi.

Harrison, Mary (1964). *A Couple's Guide to Causes and Treatments.* Houghton Mifflin Company, Boston.

Insler, V. (1981). *Some Epidemiological Aspects of Fertility Evaluation.* Elsevier North Holland, New York.

Mathur, Neeta (1989). *A Psychological Study of Infertile Women.* Ph.D. thesis in Psychology. Mohan Lal Sukhadia University, Udaipur.

Niranjana, S. (2000), *Status of Women and Family Welfare.* Kanishka Publishers Distributors, New Delhi.

Prabhu, P.N. (1963). *Hindu Social Organization.* Popular Prakashan, Mumbai.

Stevenson, Sinclair (1910). *The Rites of Twice Born.* Oxford University Press, London.

4

Social Interactions and Behaviour

India is a vast country with varying cultural and religious practices. Its diversity lies in its social and cultural variations, linguistic and region-wise different basis of formation of its social institutions. In the area of demographic behaviour in different regional and cultural settings there exists different notions about the sex preferences as well as the size of family. Invariably, the preference is shown by people for the birth of a son in the family (Niranjana, 2000).

People of India perceive children as essential to their marriage and family life. The reasons given for procreation include continuity of the family name and lineage (*kula*), or "leaving part of oneself to posterity". Reproduction is simply taken for granted as a central function of marriage. To remain deliberately childless and to admit this publicly is to invite sanctions of various kinds, which include reprimands from parents and ostracism from kin, friends and neighbours (Bardwick, 1974).

As a social institution, marriage has emerged in order to satisfy certain very basic biological, psychological and social needs of man. And, even though it has gone through many changes during the past centuries and several of its original functions like the educational, the economic, the religious and the recreational have been gradually taken away by other social and state agencies, yet its basic functions which centre around the primary bio-psycho-social needs of man have not been affected. In the opinion of Nimkoff, if there were no offsprings born, it would be improper to speak of the family, for there is no such thing as a 'childless family'; a more correct expression in such a case would be 'childless marriage' (Prabhu, 1963).

APPROACH TOWARDS CHILDLESSNESS

The couples viewed bearing and rearing of children as a confirmation of one's masculinity and femininity. Procreation, for a male, was a concrete demonstration of his virility and maturity to self and community. Begetting a child ensured his self-image as a complete man and enhanced his esteem among his peers. A man who failed in this respect would be the object of sympathy, sarcasm or ridicule, while the inability to produce a child, especially a son, was often seen as indicative of a lack of manliness. Such men were advised by friends and relatives to consult ayurvedic pandits (specialists in indigenous medicines), whose herbal medicine was believed to enhance sexual potency. It was also not uncommon for men, especially during the early years of marriage, to follow a special diet (e.g., almond milk, eggs, ghee, saffron and so on) which is believed to reinforce or enhance their virility (Arnold et al., 1975).

For women bearing children is a demonstration of their fecundity, femininity and conformity to the virtue of motherhood. Women's destiny lies mainly in her procreation; the mark of her success as a person is in her living and thriving children. In traditional joint families, begetting a son brought a woman more respect and power. A girl child on the other hand gave them fear of dowry, since it introduced uncertainty regarding their ability to successfully meet parental obligations (Mandelbaum, 1970).

People take parenthood as much for granted as birth and death—i.e., being born, getting an education, then a job, followed by marriage, parenthood and finally death. This is some kind of unwritten cosmic schedule that humans follow and no one really thinks about the progression of events as they live their lives. They just flow from one phase of life to another in a seamless fashion. For couples who discover that they cannot have children for whatever reason, the loss of parenthood, a basic ingredient of life, comes as a rude shock.

Most couples when told that they are infertile find it difficult to accept this verdict. After all, people all over the world are having a baby every minute. It is the most natural thing in the world. The next thought that occurs to them is considering the rate at which medical technology is advancing—surely the problem can be fixed. This is true to a certain extent. Various infertility treatments have worked for many couples who were having difficulty conceiving a child. But there are still some couples that slip through the cracks. After spending huge amounts of money and following all the doctors' instructions, some couples still fail to conceive a child.

Initially, the couple has a hope that after treatment, the wife will be able to conceive. After rigorous investigations, when it is found that it is very difficult or impossible to conceive, both the partners are under severe stress, and they undergo a situation of helplessness, because this stress is found to be unavoidable and they cannot do anything. This helplessness is a learned response in the face of a situation, which cannot be controlled (Mathur, 1989). Women do not construct gender identities when they cannot be mothers, in a context such as India, where strong pronatalist attitudes mandate motherhood. Making babies is how women are expected to form adult identities the world over, and in non-western 'developing' societies the gender consequences of infertility can be grave (Inhorn, 1994). Infertility has a negative social value in Indian culture. Formerly, it was viewed as a disgrace and a mark of shame. In many societies, wife often has no status until she becomes a mother. The great problems of the infertile couples are social and cultural deprivation and ignorance of sexual physiology. Due to these problems, the problems of role expectations and self-image among the couples with nervous system disorders arise which they cannot work through (Masters and Johnson, 1970).

In the present study, it was found that in those cases where the problem was diagnosed in the males, the respondents tried to hide the fact and held women responsible for childlessness. When probed, they denied the fact by saying that doctors could not diagnose the problem or the couple never went for medical examination. In other cases where females were diagnosed infertile, it was disclosed instantly. Gender difference was seen in the fact that the respondents found it easier to put the blame on women. Men's infertility was generally kept as a secret. The wives themselves actively helped to keep it a secret when husbands were diagnosed infertile. Women were blamed in those cases also where there was pregnancy wastage.

The respondents' approach towards the problem of childlessness was inferred for their responses and categorised into three types: happy, normal and tense. Overall, females were found to be more tense in their approach as compared to males. The striking emotional feelings reported by different respondents were depression, anxiety, irritability, helplessness, anger and jealousy. The emotional responses to infertility were more intense in those cases where women were diagnosed responsible and where husbands and in-laws were not supportive (see also Table 4.6).

One of the female respondent stated:

> Because of childlessness, I feel cut off, left out and feel that nobody cares for me. I feel socially isolated and emotionally disturbed because of the negative attitude of society.

A feeling of guilt was found in those cases where an organic problem was stated as a cause of childlessness. Depression was most commonly seen in case of female respondents. One of the male respondents where infertility was unexplained stated:

> My wife has given me the ultimatum that if she will not get pregnant by the end of year she will commit suicide as she wants a baby badly.

CHANGE IN INTERPERSONAL RELATIONSHIP

Infertility affects the couples in a number of ways. The females undergo a conflict over their femininity and fear of reproduction and pregnancy. A man's self-esteem is directly associated with masculinity, and that of a woman with femininity. Intact marriages are found to be associated with high self-esteem. In the case of the infertile couples, a man often suffers a loss of self-esteem when he starts analysing himself on the grounds of masculinity as a reaction to his wife's anxiety. A woman also feels this loss especially when she is found responsible for it. Being childless is taken as a severe threat to her femininity by herself. This results in an unhealthy marital relationship full of various types of inhibitions.

Although this is done out of ignorance and lack of proper knowledge, the female partner is more likely to be affected by childlessness, rather than the male partner. Her social status or prestige and acceptability in the family and society is largely determined by her fertility which in turn effects her self-image. Thus, an infertile woman has to undergo the loss of status of prestige also (Mathur, 1989).

Infertility imposes a strain on any marriage when the basic human need as parenthood is frustrated. It is a severe threat to masculinity and femininity, which leads to aggression, depression and emotional complications. The divorce rates among infertile marriages were greater than with those couples with children. Divorce rates were higher in urban areas as compared to the rural ones (Sharma, 1990).

Infertility affects the marital relationships on the aspects such as sexual identity, self-esteem, communication patterns and future life choices (Shapiro and Constance, 1982). A loss of significant relationship is an unspoken fear. Because both, man and woman are hurting, tired and under great pressure, they feel depleted of physical and emotional energy. They may become less able to fulfil each other's needs and thereby suffer a loss of closeness to the point of feeling worlds apart (Mazor, 1979).

Childlessness had a far more negative influence on the female subjects' behaviour with disappointment, jealousy and marital dissatisfaction (Brand, 1981). The husband or the wife often feels guilty thinking that it is his or her fault that conception was not possible. Sometimes the man or woman's own feelings of guilt drive them to ascribe these feelings to their partners. This is usually unwarranted as the thought may have never crossed their partners' minds, nor have they acted in a manner indicating that they blamed the other person.

The respondents, childless couples of this study were enjoying harmonious relations before diagnosis of the problem. They had good understanding, love and affection between them. After diagnosis of the problem or due to delay in pregnancy, major change in the interpersonal relations of couples was observed. They used to fight over small matters, there was lack of understanding between them and they tried to find fault in each other.

More positive interpersonal relations were also reported. Respondents stated that more love and affection developed between the couple and their relationship faced no threat as the bond between them was strong and they used to support and console each other by saying:

> Nobody can be blamed in this matter. It is the wish of God.

This was most commonly seen in those cases where males were diagnosed sterile. Where relationship turned from positive to negative, relatives reported that the couples had good interpersonal relations earlier but as the problem was diagnosed or pregnancy got delayed, the couples got depressed and felt lonely. In many cases, males used to stay out of the home for long period of time, started smoking and drinking alcohol in large quantity. This attitude gave rise to a distance between them and their relationship got worsened. These relationships were found to be more prevalent in those cases, where females were diagnosed infertile and where infertility was unexplained due to which again the blame for childlessness was indirectly placed on females.

Some respondents reported that their relations did not suffer because of infertility but had become stronger. There was no friction due to childlessness.

SOCIETAL ATTITUDE TOWARDS CHILDLESSNESS

Right from the time she is a little girl, a woman is brought up with the idea that marriage is her goal and thereafter, becoming a mother is the final legitimate destination. Most women continue to believe that this is their socially allotted role. The function of a mother is to bear children and bring them up, if necessary, as is often the case, at the expense of sacrificing and neglecting her own needs and aspirations.

Widespread but poorly documented is evidence of the severe emotional harassment experienced by large numbers of childless women in their marital homes. Harassment comes in many forms ostracism from family celebrations, taunting and stigmatisation, negative attitudes, as well as beating, withholding of food and health care. Throughout the world, adult identity for women is normatively organised around the milestone of motherhood, and the norm is particularly strong in India. To be sure, there are currents of change in the motherhood mandate with economic liberalisation, which is influencing ideas about marriage and reconfiguring family forms. Nevertheless, arranged marriage continues to be the dominant form and pronatalism remains, even if diversity is possible in the timing of marriage and childbearing, especially among India's growing middle class. While 'delay' may be tolerated, women are ultimately expected to marry and reproduce (Riessman, 2000).

Infertility is as much a state of mind as a physical disorder. Most women feel insecure about their failure and the elements of family dynamics effect the woman's desire to have children. Infertile women are often ambivalent about being cured especially after a prolonged course of painful uncomfortable and ineffective treatment (Reboul, 1982). Perception of childless women revealed it to be a negative or discreditable attitude.

Infertile couples' relatives and friends did not give genuine support in majority of the cases. Pregnant women and other people's children often evoked negative feelings among them (Lalos et al., 1986).

In the present study, during the early years of marriage, the female respondents reported that their family members and relatives were more loving, cooperative and understanding but as the problem was diagnosed, they observed a change in their relationship. It was reported by female respondents that their family members had become quarrelsome, frustrated over small matters and husband had increased alcohol intake and used to stay out of home for a comparatively increased duration. In some cases they avoided their wife's company.

It was evident from the responses that fertility or ability to produce children has a positive social value. Family and society looks down upon the couples who are not able to bear children. Insensitive behaviour to their childlessness was targeted by their family members, neighbours, relatives and friends. They were under constant social pressure from family and society and some females even had to face the threat of remarriage and divorce. Because of such attitudes the childless couples especially women felt isolated from family and society; they expressed the feeling of being excluded from couples having children at family gathering and other social events. Men also reported the feeling of isolation but women reported greater social isolation especially in those cases where family members were not supporting them.

It was also found that parents have a positive and sympathetic attitude towards the problem faced by childless couples. Respondents stated that they were understanding and cooperative. They understood the couple and their feelings very well and tried to avoid such circumstances, which could hurt their feelings. They neither made demands on the couple to bear a child, nor criticised the behaviour of the affected couple. Whenever the affected couple got depressed or felt isolated, they tried to console and encourage by saying such words as:

> "Have faith in God", "God will help you one day", "Believe in God, everything will be alright."

BEHAVIOURAL CHANGES IN CHILDLESS COUPLES

When a couple hopes of becoming parents, they in a way are very strongly attached to their unborn child. However, when the hope disappears declaring their inability to conceive and after giving a feeling of disappointment and it is so painful that a tendency to deny the facts develops. They feel depleted of the emotional energy. Self-directed, self-controlled and hard working people are devastated by the experience of infertility. They may undergo a trauma depending upon individual characteristics. There is a far more negative influence over the females as they are thought to be responsible for childlessness. They show jealousy and marital dissatisfaction. They have a lower level of satisfaction. The infertile women experience and confront the ambiguity about their infertility and treatment.

Women who are infertile often feel that the fact that they cannot bear children makes them less of a woman or inadequate in some way. Unfortunately, this is a sentiment that is often supported in society. Being barren is not a stigma that a woman should have to bear like a cross for the rest of her life. There is much more to a woman than her ability to bear child. Similarly, if conception was not possible as a result of male infertility, the male partner may feel that it is a slur on his manhood.

The infertile individuals may undergo a loss of relationship, health, status, prestige, self-esteem, self-confidence, security, fantasy and loss of something or someone of great symbolic value (White and David, 1977). There was deterioration of emotional disturbances as well (Walker, 1978). Childless couples react overtly with a feeling of disappointment. Initially, the prevailing of infertility may be so painful that there may be a tendency to deny the fact (Wiche, 1976).

In the infertile couples emotional reactions were found, such as sadness, depression, anger, confusion, desperation, hurt, embarrassment and humiliation. Behavioural reactions to infertility include disorganisation, destructibility, exhaustion, moodiness and obsessive thought and behaviour. According to a report, Buganda has a high incidence of infertility. There are efforts being made to reduce the social consequences of infertility as it imposes serious emotional effects on an infertile woman (Bennett, 1965).

It was also found that most of the childless couples had a favourable attitude to other people's children and they liked being in their company. Among the couples where husbands experienced impotency, the women showed anger towards the husband, there were psychiatric symptoms and dreams about their concern for the husband, a wish to be rid of him and a guilt over this wish (Berger, 1980).

In the present study, most of the respondents reported withdrawal from several social activities that reminded them of their inability to conceive. They stopped attending the social gathering where they were reproached of their infertility. One of the respondents stated:

> I never go for birthday parties of children.

They also tried to withdraw from the thought of children and tried not to think about infertility consciously. Many of female respondents who remained depressed and frustrated because of their infertility stated that they cried many times whenever they thought about their infertility or whenever somebody reminded them or hurt their feelings by passing comments, remarks and taunts. For them crying served as a form of relief.

Many of male and female respondents were suffering in silence about their infertility. They believed that it was God's will that they remained childless; as they could not do anything against God's will so they decided they would suffer in silence.

Respondents were asked to tell about their reactions on getting news about pregnancy of some relatives, friends or neighbours. More females as compared to male respondents showed negative responses on hearing this kind of news. They reported feelings of annoyance, jealousy, misfortune and failure. Some of the respondents stated:

> It seems that world is full of pregnant ladies. I feel so jealous about the women who successfully conceive especially when they do not want the baby. At the time I become so jealous and curse my luck.

Another respondent reported:

> When I see that my friends or my husband's friends of the same age group go through the experience of pregnancy and satisfaction of parenthood, I feel incomplete and depressed.

Another respondent stated:

> I avoid congratulating or meeting the friends or relatives, who are pregnant or become parents. It does not mean that I am not happy or I am jealous but I am afraid that I might start crying.

However, some of the respondents also had positive feelings towards pregnancy of others and they consider them as lucky because they are complete and they will not face the psycho-social repercussions of childlessness. They felt happy about pregnancy of others.

It was found that men often tried to approach other people's children, which mostly belonged to his family, while women avoided them. Adverse feelings towards relative's children were very common among the infertile women. Most of the infertile couples, particularly the men often find it difficult to talk to others about their childlessness.

Childless couples were asked to delineate whether they were invited to social and religious functions, their reaction towards participation in such functions and the reason for not attending such functions. It was found that some of the female respondents themselves avoided attending such ceremonies because they felt embarrassed and humiliated on such occasions, as people around them passed some remarks or the other and they became the topic for gossip and conversation. Some of respondents stated that they were not invited on birthday parties of children, as they did not have children and they knew it very well that participation of childless females in social gatherings, especially rituals related to pregnancy or childbirth was restricted because these women were considered inauspicious or incomplete. They were called only at the time of having food but not invited at the time of performance of rituals.

Childless males as such did not report any negative reactions for such ceremonies and rituals. It is perhaps because these ceremonies are more female centred and where males did not have many roles to perform.

EFFECT OF CHILDLESSNESS ON THE TENSIONS OF MARRIED LIFE OF THE COUPLE

An attempt was made to study the attitude of the spouses towards each other and the effect of this attitude on their married life, due to childlessness. Marital relationships have been divided into seven stages, struggle and intimacy being the two extremes (Table 4.1). Thus, the marital relationships have neither been found to be too full of conflicts or struggles nor too intimate. One-fourth of the couples have reported their lives to be completely indifferent whereas nearly 25 per cent couples were falling into conflicts and tense life. About 23 per cent have agreed upon a tension-free relationship and 24.2 per cent couples maintain a cordial relationship.

The feeling of struggle has mostly been found in the urban slums where 34.5 per cent couples quarrel among themselves due to childlessness.

Most of the villagers talk about tension-free and cordial relationships. Only 50 per cent couples out of those who have been married for less than three years have the behaviour of struggle and conflicts relationship. Struggles and conflicts were mostly found in couples falling in the scheduled tribes category, which was more than 11 per cent. One-third of couples in the general category maintain cordial relationships.

None of the couples, whose men are working (services), show a conflict and struggle in their married life; on the contrary, 31 per cent couples have shown a cordial relationship. The occupation of women also affects the married life and behaviour. This is made clear because 32 per cent women having a business of their own, have a cordial relationship with their husbands and only 4 per cent of such women have a struggle in their relationships.

Conflicts and struggles have not been found in couples out of love marriage, but there has been a tension in the relationship. In their case, 21 per cent couples remain tensed,

Table 4.1

Effect of Childlessness on the Tensions of Married Life of Couples Percentage Distribution of Couples by Selected Background Characteristics

Characteristics	*Conflicts & Struggle*	*Tension*	*Avoidance*	*Indifferent*	*Tension-free*	*Cordial*	*Intimacy*	*Total Per cent*	*Number*	x^2 *Value/ df and Significance*
Residence										
Rural	2.30	10.00	5.70	23.90	30.70	27.40	0.00	100.00	88	
Urban slums	34.50	0.00	6.90	17.20	6.90	20.70	13.80	100.00	29	66.396/12**
Urban	1.60	12.20	7.30	26.00	22.00	22.80	8.10	100.00	123	
Duration of Marriage										
<3	0.00	50.00	0.00	0.00	50.00	0.00	0.00	100.00	4	
3-8	5.20	6.20	12.40	9.30	16.50	42.20	8.20	100.00	97	
8-13	2.90	11.80	4.10	33.80	32.40	12.10	2.90	100.00	68	94.765/24**
13-18	22.60	19.40	0.00	19.40	19.40	9.50	9.70	100.00	31	
18+	0.00	5.00	2.50	50.00	25.00	15.00	2.50	100.00	40	
Caste										
General	6.70	10.00	5.00	16.70	25.00	31.60	5.00	100.00	60	
SC	3.30	1.70	13.30	20.00	31.70	23.30	6.70	100.00	60	
ST	11.70	8.30	3.30	30.00	16.70	21.70	8.30	100.00	60	32.065/18*
OBC	1.70	20.00	5.00	30.00	20.00	20.00	3.30	100.00	60	

Contd...

Contd...										
Husband's Occupation										
Own business	3.80	11.40	12.70	24.10	16.50	22.80	8.70	100.00	79	
Service	0.00	10.20	4.60	24.10	24.10	30.60	6.40	100.00	108	47.089/12**
Agriculture	20.80	7.50	1.90	24.50	32.10	13.20	0.00	100.00	53	
Wife's Occupation										
Own business	4.00	8.00	4.00	20.00	16.00	32.00	16.00	100.00	25	
Service	3.60	7.30	10.90	20.00	16.40	29.10	12.70	100.00	55	40.598/18**
Agriculture	19.40	3.20	0.00	16.10	38.70	22.60	0.00	100.00	31	
Housewife	3.90	13.20	7.00	28.70	23.30	21.70	2.20	100.00	129	
Type of Marriage										
Love marriage	0.00	21.20	0.00	3.00	6.10	48.50	21.20	100.00	33	
Arranged marriage	6.80	8.20	7.70	27.50	26.10	20.30	3.40	100.00	207	46.433/6**
Total	5.80	10.00	6.70	24.20	23.30	24.20	5.80	100.00	240	

* Chi-square is significant at the 0.05 level.

** Chi-square is significant at the 0.01 level.

whereas 26 per cent couples out of arranged marriages run their families without any tension. The nature of residence, period of marriage, caste, occupational status of the husband and wife and the kind of marriage are associated with several aspects of conflict and tension. The Chi-square test shows significant difference at .01 and .05 level.

Apart from this, significance was also tested on the basis of the kind of house (*kachcha*, semi-*pucca, pucca*) and the nature of family but no significant difference was observed.

RESPONSE TO CHILDLESSNESS

Table 4.2 shows that the reactions of men and women are different on their knowing that they are responsible for childlessness. When the thought-process of men was studied, it was found that only 16 per cent men attribute it to fate, whereas 67 per cent women hold their fate/destiny responsible. A large number of women greatly believe in the theory of childlessness due to sins in the earlier birth. It was found that 48 per cent women believe childlessness is the fruit of those sins committed in earlier birth. Women also believe that this childlessness may also have been caused due to some curse on them, but men call this a superstition and only 10 per cent of them support this view of women. Considering childlessness as the will of God is also a major part of the beliefs of women and was reported by

Table 4.2

Reactions After Realising the Responsibility for Childlessness

Reactions	*Female*		*Male*	
	Frequency	*Per cent*	*Frequency*	*Per cent*
Fate	162	67.50	39	16.30
Sins of earlier work	115	47.90	26	10.80
Curse	106	44.20	26	10.80
God's will	183	76.30	48	20.00

more than three-fourths of the female population. Comparatively, this belief that "childlessness is the will of God" is greater in men, but such men are only one-fifth of the male population.

It may be concluded that as compared to men, women greatly believe in the fruits of their acts in the previous birth, curse and fate, whereas men have a greater belief in the will of God.

REACTIONS TO THE INABILITY OF SPOUSE

Table 4.3 has been made to indicate the reactions on knowing that one's life partner is responsible for childlessness. This table reveals that a woman not only faces cruelty in the society when she herself is responsible, but also when her husband is the one with the fault and she has to face adverse situations in the family and society. Whereas 67 per cent women owe their childlessness to their fate (Table 4.2), only 16 per cent blame it on their fate even when they know that the fault is with their husbands. An entirely contrary behaviour can be seen in the case of men. Only 16.3 per cent blame their fate when they themselves are responsible for childlessness, whereas when their wives are at fault, more than 50 per cent of them blame their fate for having married such a woman and being childless. Acceptance of childlessness on the basis of beliefs like the result of sins made in the earlier birth, curse or the will of God is greater in women. The inability of men to produce a child or

Table 4.3
Reactions to the Inability of Spouse for Childlessness

Reactions	*Female*		*Male*	
	Frequency	*Per cent*	*Frequency*	*Per cent*
Fate	38	15.80	121	50.40
Sins of earlier work	26	10.80	104	43.30
Curse	28	11.70	93	38.80
God's will	45	18.80	186	77.50

the realisation of being responsible for childlessness hurts their ego. May be, this is the reason why only 11 per cent men (Table 4.2) believe that it is the result of the sins of their earlier birth. Whereas, when the inability is found in their wives, around 43 per cent of men believe that it is the result of the sins of the earlier birth that they have to repay now in the form of childlessness.

WIFE HOLDS HUSBAND RESPONSIBLE FOR CHILDLESSNESS

More than half of the men who are responsible for childlessness disagree that their wives consider them responsible for it (Table 4.4). Around 16 per cent men accept that their wives often keep mentioning about it; the maximum percentage (38%) was found in urban slums. More than half of the men in *pucca* houses state that their wives have never told them that they are responsible for the childlessness.

On the one hand, where 26.7 per cent men belonging to the scheduled tribes category have stated that they are made to realise their responsibility of childlessness, time and again by their wives, about three-fourths of men belonging to the general category never have to face such a situation.

Among the men who are engaged in agriculture, about 32.1 per cent, of their wives express sadness over childlessness due to a fault in their husbands and therefore remind them of their being responsible over and over again. The number of wives holding husbands responsible for childlessness is greater in arranged marriages as compared to love marriages.

HUSBAND HOLDS WIFE RESPONSIBLE FOR CHILDLESSNESS

When childless women were questioned about their husbands holding them responsible for childlessness (Table 4.5), around 50 per cent women accept that their husbands never make them realise about them being responsible for it. About 19 per cent

Table 4.4
Wife Holds Husband Responsible for Childlessness
Percentage Distribution of Couples by Selected Background Characteristics

Characteristics	*Often*	*Some-times in Anger*	*Uncon-sciously*	*Never*	*Total Per cent*	*Number*	*x^2 Value/ df and Significance*
Residence							
Rural	14.80	14.80	20.40	50.00	100.00	88	
Urban slums	37.90	13.80	13.80	34.50	100.00	29	13.981/6*
Urban	12.20	18.70	13.80	55.30	100.00	123	
House							
Kachcha	25.00	8.30	18.80	47.90	100.00	48	
Semi-pucca	22.50	18.30	16.90	42.30	100.00	71	12.682/6*
Pucca	9.10	19.00	14.90	57.00	100.00	121	
Caste							
General	15.00	1.70	10.00	73.30	100.00	60	
SC	8.30	18.30	28.40	45.00	100.00	60	42.515/9**
ST	26.70	28.30	3.30	41.70	100.00	60	
OBC	15.00	18.30	23.40	43.30	100.00	60	
Husband's Occupation							
Own business	19.00	20.30	7.60	53.10	100.00	79	
Service	6.50	11.10	22.20	60.20	100.00	108	31.88/6**
Agriculture	32.10	22.60	17.00	28.30	100.00	53	
Type of Marriage							
Love marriage	9.10	9.10	6.10	75.70	100.00	33	9.645/3*
Arranged marriage	17.40	17.90	17.90	46.80	100.00	207	
Total	16.30	16.70	16.20	50.80	100.00	240	

* Chi-square is significant at the 0.05 level.
** Chi-square is significant at the 0.01 level.

women state that sometimes in anger their husbands do make them realise their fault. According to 38 per cent women living in urban slums, their husbands constantly hold them responsible for childlessness, whereas, this percentage is nearly 10 per cent in urban women; education and the urban effect are observed as the underlined reasons. Also, 60 per cent women, out of the couples living in *pucca* houses are never held responsible for childlessness The highest percentage (about 28), is of those husbands belonging to the scheduled tribes who, sometimes in anger, make their wives realise their responsibility for childlessness.

Table 4.5

Husband Holds Wife Responsible for Childlessness
Percentage Distribution of Couples by Selected Background Characteristics

Characteristics	*Often*	*Sometimes in Anger*	*Unconsciously*	*Never*	*Total Per cent*	*Number*	*x^2 Value/ df and Significant*
Residence							
Rural	12.50	14.80	27.20	45.50	100.00	88	
Urban slums	37.90	13.80	13.80	34.50	100.00	29	22.657/6**
Urban	9.80	20.30	13.80	56.10	100.00	123	
House							
Kachcha	25.00	8.30	18.80	47.90	100.00	48	
Semi-pucca	22.50	18.30	25.40	33.80	100.00	71	26.364/6**
Pucca	5.00	20.70	14.80	59.50	100.00	121	
Caste							
General	10.00	1.70	20.00	68.30	100.00	60	
SC	8.30	18.30	28.40	45.00	100.00	60	46.512/9**
ST	26.70	28.30	3.30	41.70	100.00	60	
OBC	11.70	21.70	23.30	43.30	100.00	60	
Husband's Occupation							
Own business	13.90	22.80	7.60	55.70	100.00	79	
Service	6.50	11.10	27.80	54.60	100.00	108	33.887/6**
Agriculture	30.20	22.60	17.00	30.20	100.00	53	
Wife's Occupation							
Own business	8.00	4.00	28.00	60.00	100.00	25	
Service	5.50	21.80	7.20	65.50	100.00	55	23.449/9**
Agriculture	25.80	16.10	29.10	29.00	100.00	31	
Housewife	16.80	18.60	18.90	45.70	100.00	129	
Total	14.20	17.50	18.70	49.60	100.00	240	

* Chi-square is significant at the 0.05 level.
** Chi-square is significant at the 0.01 level.

Around 30 per cent men, engaged in agricultural jobs, make their wives realise their responsibility for childlessness and if the women are also engaged in agricultural jobs, their percentage falls down to 26 per cent. Out of the women engaged in services, the husbands of about 65 per cent of them never held them responsible. Thus, a significant relationship has been found between occupation and behaviour.

A significant difference was found in the behaviour of husbands and wives on the basis of their occupational status. Significant difference was also found on the grounds of residence, kinds of house and caste.

COMPARISON OF THE BEHAVIOUR OF MEN AND WOMEN

Table 4.6 indicates the comparative study conducted on the changes in the behaviour of men and women due to childlessness. The behaviour of a man and a woman varies on different occasions. The variation in behaviour is due to many reasons. The study of behaviours was conducted mainly on six points. On being invited to a child's birthday party, 50 per cent men have a normal behaviour and 39 per cent men feel happy. Whereas only around one-third women are able to be normal;

Table 4.6

Comparative Behaviour Patterns

Percentage Distribution of Couples by Selected Background Characteristics

Behaviour/Feelings	*Male*			*Female*		
	Happy	*Normal*	*Tense*	*Happy*	*Normal*	*Tense*
Invited to a child's birthday	38.80	49.60	11.70	18.30	32.50	49.20
Seeing a pregnant woman	26.70	63.70	9.60	17.50	37.10	45.40
Seeing the toys or clothes of a child	40.40	52.10	7.50	26.70	32.90	40.40
Seeing children in films or on TV	48.30	44.20	7.50	32.90	27.90	39.20
Seeing children of family members	65.00	22.90	12.10	27.90	11.70	60.40
Invited to an auspicious occasion	60.00	28.30	11.70	23.80	15.00	61.30

50 per cent women become tensed. They fail to hide the grief of childlessness and so refuse to attend those birthday parties.

It has also been observed that even when the inability is in the men, 63.7 per cent of them behave normally on seeing a pregnant woman, whereas 45.4 per cent women feel jealous and this leads to sorrow and tenseness. The behaviour of men and women also vary when they see the toys or clothes of a child. About 52 per cent men feel normal and 40.4 per cent feel happy. On the other hand, 40 per cent childless women become sad and tense. The difference in the behaviour of men and women has also been observed due to a difference in their basic natures. Women are more sensitive and consider their womanhood assured through motherhood. That is why, when they see children in films or on their television sets, 40 per cent of them fail to control their emotions and thus become tense. Contrary to this, because men are always engaged in miscellaneous activities, TV or films have no significant effect on their emotions; only 7.5 per cent men are influenced by TV or films. Even when there are many children in the house, female still longs for a child of her own. This kind of possessive mentality does not allow her to maintain a normal behaviour towards other children in the family. It was seen that 60 per cent women express this behaviour in the form of tension. On the other hand, 65 per cent men are normal with other children in the house and thus remain happy with them.

In the transition period of the society, the attitude towards childlessness is also changing. A trend of optional childlessness has also been noticed in urban places. The practice named as DINKs "Double income, No kids" is spreading rapidly in metropolitan cities. But at the same time, not much change has been observed in the mentality towards the inability of a woman to produce a child. Especially in our study area, 'barrenness' is a stigma for women. Most of the women (61%), hesitate to attend an auspicious occasion, only 23.8 per cent women feel happy to do so. Opposite to this, 60 per cent men show happiness to attend any auspicious occasion, because the stigma of childlessness is not a hindrance for men. Regardless of who is unable to produce a child, mainly the women are looked down upon by the society.

BEHAVIOUR PROBLEMS OF MEN AND WOMEN

The behaviour of men and women with respect to various circumstances has been studied on six scale items with three responses: happy, normal and tense (score: 1, 2, 3). The mean score for male and female is shown in Table 4.7. On being invited to a child's birthday party, the attitude of male ranges from that of happiness to normal. Similarly, on seeing pregnant women or on looking at the toys and clothes of children, their behaviour does not become tense. On the contrary, women feel tense on attending a child's birthday party and the same feeling arises when they see a pregnant woman. A great difference in the behaviour of men and women has been observed when they see a child of their relatives or on being invited to any special occasion. Whereas men feel happy, women are generally tense. In the same way, men have a normal or a happy behaviour on being invited for a special occasion.

Table 4.7
Mean Table of Behavioural Patterns

Behaviour/Feelings	*Male*	*Female*
Invited to a child's birthday	1.72	2.30
Seeing a pregnant woman	1.82	2.27
Seeing the toys or clothes of a child	1.67	2.13
Seeing children in films or on TV	1.59	2.06
Seeing children of family members	1.47	2.32
Invited to an auspicious occasion	1.51	2.37

EFFECT OF BACKGROUND CHARACTERISTICS ON CONFLICTS AND TENSION IN HUSBAND-WIFE RELATIONSHIP

The respondents were asked about their mutual relationship, to see the effect of childlessness on married life. One factor was formed by combining the responses which included variables—

conflict, tension, avoidance and indifference and named "conflicts and avoidance". Tension free, cordial and intimacy form another factor—'cordiality'. The first factor is analysed in detail.

It is found that age of the female, male and duration of marriage have a great impact on the husband-wife relationship. Along with this, type of family, husband's occupation and wife's occupational status are deeply related to conflict or tensions between husband and wife.

People residing in urban slums and in semi-*pucca* houses have more conflict and avoidance behaviour. When the female crosses the age of 40 years, her reproduction capacity is severely decreased, then the conflict and avoidance is found to be greater between husband and wife.

Conflict is found to be least when the husband's age group in between 25 to 29 years. Maximum conflict and avoidance is found in Other Backward Classes (OBC) category. When relationship was analysed on the basis of type of marriage, it was found that conflict is lesser in love marriages. The husbands, who are in service, have better relations with their wife than those husbands who are engaged in agriculture.

On the basis of rural and urban settings, no significant difference was found. Only one-third women in urban slums are such who never made their husbands realise about this problem. Duration of marriage also influences the behaviour of a wife. Therefore, in couples married for less than three years, only 50 per cent wives hold their husbands responsible. Whereas in couples married for three to eight years, more than 60 per cent females are such who never held their husbands responsible (Table 4.8).

It was clarified earlier also that maximum conflict is found in OBC category. Along with these only 40 per cent females are such who never held their husbands responsible for childlessness. Type of family, occupational status of wife and income also influence various behaviours of wife. As many as 80 per cent wives of families having income of

Table 4.8
Social Interactions and Behaviours
Percentage Distribution of Couples by Selected Background Characteristics

Characteristics	*Conflicts and Avoidance*	*Wife Never Holds Husband Responsible*	*Husband Never Holds Wife Responsible*	*Number*
Residence	*	*	**	
Rural	41.90	50.00	45.50	88
Urban slums	58.60	34.50	34.50	29
Urban	47.10	55.30	56.10	123
House		*	**	
Kachcha	43.80	47.90	47.90	48
Semi-pucca	61.10	42.30	33.80	71
Pucca	44.60	57.00	59.50	121
Current Age	**			
19-24	38.90	57.40	59.30	54
25-29	45.80	45.80	47.00	83
30-34	47.00	47.10	49.00	51
35-39	33.40	44.40	44.40	18
40+	73.30	46.70	46.70	34
Husband's Age	**		*	
19-24	50.00	66.70	66.70	6
25-29	26.30	57.90	59.60	57
30-34	50.70	45.30	42.70	75
35-39	56.20	43.90	50.90	57
40+	53.30	57.10	57.10	14
Duration of Marriage	**	**	**	
<3	50.00	50.00	50.00	4
3-8	33.10	61.90	64.90	97
8-13	52.90	42.60	42.60	68
13-18	61.40	22.60	22.60	31
18+	57.50	60.00	45.00	40
Caste	*	*	**	
General	38.40	73.30	68.30	60
SC	38.30	45.00	45.00	60

Contd...

Contd...

ST	53.30	41.70	41.70	60
OBC	56.70	43.30	43.30	60
Family	**	*	**	
Nuclear	42.70	50.30	46.20	143
Joint	52.60	66.10	69.60	97
Husband's Occupation	**	**	**	
Own business	52.00	53.20	55.70	79
Service	38.90	60.20	54.60	108
Agriculture	54.70	28.30	30.20	53
Wife's Occupation	**	*	**	
Own business	36.00	60.00	60.00	25
Service	41.80	63.60	65.50	55
Agriculture	38.70	29.00	29.00	31
Housewife	52.80	48.80	45.70	129
Monthly Income	**	*	**	
<2000	44.40	37.50	37.50	36
2000-5000	48.40	50.80	45.10	124
5000-8000	23.90	71.40	71.40	42
8000-11000	0.00	40.00	100.00	10
11000+	20.00	80.00	85.00	28
Type of Marriage	**	*	*	
Love marriage	24.20	75.80	75.80	33
Arranged marriage	50.20	46.90	45.40	207
Total				240

* Chi-square is significant at the 0.05 level.
** Chi-square is significant at the 0.01 level.

more than Rs 11,000 per month do not hold their husbands responsible.

The analysis of the behaviour of husbands where wives are responsible for childlessness does not reveal significant difference by the type of residence unlike slums where both husband and wife hold the responsibility on each other for childlessness. No significant difference was found by the age of husband and wife.

In nuclear families, less family pressure was seen; that is why husband and wife hold more responsibility in each other as compared to joint families.

It is inferred that couples residing in slums, semi-*pucca* houses and earning less than Rs 5,000 per month reveal maximum conflict and avoidance behaviour in their families. Among OBC families where more conflict is noticed, they hold each other responsible for childlessness. Where females are engaged in service, less conflict was found and relations with each other were cordial. They generally do not hold each other responsible for childlessness.

SUMMARY

The couples viewed bearing and rearing children as a confirmation of one's masculinity and femininity. Procreation, for a male, was a concrete demonstration of his virility and maturity to self and community. For women, bearing children is a demonstration of their fecundity, femininity and conformity to the virtue of motherhood. It was found that in those cases where the problem was diagnosed in the males, the respondents tried to hide the fact and held women responsible for childlessness. Significant gender difference was seen in the responses of males and females.

It was found that in slums, couples residing in semi-*pucca* houses and earning less than Rs 5,000 monthly, had maximum conflicts and avoidance in their families. In OBC families, where on one hand more conflict was found on the other hand they held each other responsible for childlessness openly. In families where females were in service, less conflict was found and relations with each other were cordial. They did not hold each other responsible for childlessness.

Infertility affects the marital relationships on aspects such as sexual identity, self-esteem, and communication patterns and future life choices. It was found that age of the female, male and duration of marriage have a great impact on the husband-wife relationship. After diagnosis of the problem, major change in the interpersonal relations of couples was observed. During the early years of marriage, the female respondents reported that their family members and relatives were more loving, cooperative and understanding; but as the problem was diagnosed, they observed a change in their relationship. Significant association was found between the occupation of husband and wife, duration of marriage, residence and type of family with conflict and avoidance behaviour. Most of the respondents stated withdrawal from people and activities that reminded them of their inability to conceive. The female respondents themselves avoided attending social ceremonies because people around them passed some sarcastic remarks.

References

Arnold, Fred et al. (1975). *The Value of Children: A Cross National Study.* East West Population Institute, Honolulu.

Bardwick, J. (1974). *Evolution and Parenting Journal of Social Issues.*

Bennett, F.J. (1965). The Social, Cultural and Emotional Aspects of Sterility in Women in Buganda. *American Journal of Fertility and Sterility.*

Berger, D. (1980). Psychological Assessment of the Infertile Couples. *American Journal of Psychiatry.*

Brand, H.J. (1981). The Influence of Sex Difference on the Acceptance of Infertility. *South African Journal of Psychology.*

Inhorn, Marcia C. (1994). *Quest for Conception: Gender, Infertility, and Egyptian Medical Traditions.* University of Pennsylvania Press, Philadelphia.

Lalos, A. et al. (1986). The Wish to Have a Child: A Pilot Study of the Infertile Couples. *Acta Psychiatrica Scandinavica.*

Mandelbaum, David G. (1970). *Society in India.* University of California Press, Berkeley.

Masters, W.H. and Johnson, V.E. (1970). *Human Sexual Inadequacy.* Little Brown, Boston.

Mathur, Neeta (1989). *A Psychological Study of Infertile Women.* Ph.D. thesis in Psychology. Mohan Lal Sukhadia University, Udaipur.

Mazor, M.D. (1979). Barren Couples. *Psychology Today.*

Miall, C.E. (1985). The Stigma of Involuntarily Childlessness. *Social Problems.*

Niranjana, S. (2000). Marriage and Child Bearing Practices. *Study of Women and Family Behaviour.* Kanishka Publishers and Distributors, New Delhi.

Prabhu, P.N. (1963). *The Family Hindu Social Organization.* Popular Prakashan, Mumbai.

Reboul, J. (1982). Psychogenic Sterility is Dead: Let us Talk About Infertile Women. *Psychological Abstracts.*

Riessman, Catherine Kohler (2000). Stigma and Everyday Resistance Practices: Childless Women in South India. *Gender and Society.*

Shapiro, D.H. and Constance, H. (1982). The Impact of Infertility in the Marital Relationship. *Social Casework.*

Sharma, S.P. (1990). *Childlessness: Bane or Boon.* Women's Era. July (Second).

Walker, H.E. (1978). Psychiatric Aspects Infertility. *Urol. Clin. North America.*

White, R.B. and David (1977). Psychodynamics of Depression. Clinical, Biological and Psychological Perspectives. *Journal of Fertility and Sterility.*

Wiche, V.R. (1979). Psychological Reactions to Infertility. *Psychological Abstracts.*

5

Medical Assistance and Treatment

During the past few years, as research has evolved, the medical profession has gained a remarkable understanding regarding the intricacies of how a baby is conceived. There has been an explosion of new techniques for overcoming infertility and an unprecedented rush of would-be-parents to take advantage of them. Today, virtually every aspect of the reproductive cycle can be manipulated.

According to the WHO studies, the prevalence of primary and secondary infertility in India is 3 per cent and 8 per cent respectively. In Rajasthan 4.3 per cent of currently married women are infecund as per findings of the National Family Health Survey (1998-99). Couples can be childless either because of failure to conceive, pregnancy-loss or infant deaths. In the community, a derogatory term is used to refer to such women: *banjhari* or barren woman. Infertile women resort to a variety of remedies in a situation where rational therapy is as scarce as it is expensive (ARTH, 2001).

In most families, when childlessness is a problem, the wife is the first to present herself to the physician. At this initial visit, a complete history is indicated, with special attention given to menstrual function and past illnesses, which may have affected any of the genital structure. However, unless some obvious causative factor is immediately apparent in the wife, further study should await evaluation of the fertility of the husband. There still are too many instances where the wife is subjected to extensive studies without any preliminary attention to the fertility status of the husband. In Indian society, husbands do not wish to get themselves examined first for childlessness (Williams, 1964).

It was also found that some of the couples never went to medical examination although they were worried about the problem. In some cases, wives got them medically examined but the husbands did not agree for medical check up. One respondent stated:

> My mother conceived after 14 years of marriage, sisters conceived after 10 years of marriage and I am sure that I will also conceive after few years, so there is no need for medical check up.

For them the period of infertility was the waiting period because they were sure that they would conceive and so they would wait endlessly for the expected conception.

The advent of a child, particularly the first one, launches the married couple on a new career in the living routine, social roles and marital relationship. Almost all the married couples want to have children of their own. There are no absolute norms or criteria of suitability for marriage. Fitness for marriage implies the ability to meet the necessary requirements or purpose.

BIOLOGICAL FACTORS

Biologically, the object of marriage is not to legalise sexual union, but rather to ensure the survival of the species and the race. From this point of view, marriage is not merely a sexual relationship, but a parental association also. Marriage is also an union of male and female for the production and care of the offspring, and reproduction is, therefore, another fundamental objective of marriage (Mathur, 1989).

Infertility is involuntary childlessness. A couple wants to have a child and cannot conceive in spite of all their efforts. This does not mean that their problem is simply not achieving a pregnancy the first time they try. According to the standard medical definition, they will be diagnosed as infertile when the woman does not become pregnant after a year of intercourse without contraception. One full year! Twelve months of trying—and not succeeding. Twelve menstrual periods that come so regularly that they are literally a 'curse', a constant reminder of failure. Making love loses its joy. And no one seems to understand. There are many myths and misunderstandings about infertility in Indian society (Harrison, 1964).

Infertility is not a rare condition. When couples discover their infertility, they feel alone. Newspapers and television constantly remind them of the problems of overpopulation. Their friends seem either to be pregnant or to be avoiding another pregnancy. Their problem seems unique to them.

Infertility is not just a 'woman's disease'. The popular notion that the woman is always the barren partner is deeply imbedded in the society. In more recent history, rulers have given up their wives if they did not become pregnant. Even today, in most cases of infertility, it is the woman who seeks help first. But the condition is not confined to women (Harrison, 1964).

Childlessness is not confined to one particular group. Any person of childbearing age can encounter the problem. An infertile person can come from any social or economic class, from any race or religion. There is no distinct profile of the infertile person. This is a couple's problem. Two individual systems must each be working correctly before they can work together successfully to create a child.

MEDICAL ASSISTANCE

In case of unexplained childlessness, respondents consult medical experts ranging from simple physicians to infertility experts. They also visit outstation clinics for better medical treatment and expertise. There are occasions when patients may travel many miles to renowned medical centres. The investigation of infertility problems has now become so common that many patients can be treated in their own local areas. No fundamental reason is there, why a physician who is in general practice cannot do a very good job in this regard. Of course, there are special tests in infertility studies, which may require the specialist. But very often these tests are not necessary.

Most universities and teaching hospitals have infertility clinics, which are generally associated with the departments of obstetrics and gynaecology and run by doctors with a particular interest and expertise in infertility, usually subspecialists in infertility. They are also the training group for future subspecialists in infertility.

These clinics have the advantage of providing the couples with a host of doctors interested in infertility. Because they are located within a hospital, they provide them with easy access to specialists in other related fields, such as urology, endocrinology and radiology. They also have the added advantage of almost always being open to all patients, regardless of their economics situation. Some of these clinics have a sliding scale of fees that makes treatment available for almost everyone.

Another matter that is somewhat controversial must also be considered. When childless patients visit the physician, they often have in mind only one question: "Why can't we have children?" They should have two questions in mind: "Are we fit to have children? If so, why can't we?" Clearly, many couples who come to the physician should not, for one reason or another, have children. These couples may include patients with hypertension, or perhaps diabetes, and certainly they should be forewarned about the hazards of a pregnancy (Tyler, 1961).

The couples as an important milestone in their lives perceived parenthood, and they regarded decisions concerning the timing and number of children as having a far-reaching impact on their lives. Apart from social pressure, the couples' motivation to become parents shaped their decisions to enter parenthood as soon as they could or when circumstances allowed. Hardly any of the couples even remotely considered remaining childless (Ramu, 1988).

REACTIONS ABOUT THE DIAGNOSIS

Immediate reaction about the diagnosis of infertility in such respondents was studied and it was found that almost all the respondents reported going through a stage of denial. For them it was difficult to accept that this could happen to them.

One of the respondents stated:

> When I came to know about my infertility I was so shocked that I didn't have any energy and could not get out of the bed for couple of days.

Some reported that they did not feel like eating or talking to anybody and suffered in silence. They denied the fact and had the feeling that:

> This could not happen to us. The doctors must have been mistaken.

Many childless female respondents found it difficult to reveal about medical confirmation to their husbands and in-laws, as they were afraid of serious consequences. Male respondents also had the feeling of depression and shock when they heard about the inability of their wives to produce a baby. They became angry and shouted at their wives. In other cases, where males were diagnosed infertile they could not believe it and got very much disappointed. One of the male respondents stated:

I could not accept the fact because we always dream about a child and it was a shock for me to know that I could not produce one.

ALTERNATIVE THERAPIES

Many respondents believe that medical treatment works only "If one had good luck and if God wanted to give child to someone". Respondents also take Ayurvedic medicines. One particular Ayurvedic medicine known as 'Jaddi' (Root of a very rare plant) was very commonly taken by the respondents. These respondents also try other Ayurvedic medicines given by saints, pandits or traditional healer. Wherever such persons were available, respondents try to reach there.

Along with medical treatment respondents try non-medical treatment that includes consulting astrologers, saints, magico-spiritual healers, visiting various shrines, following religious practices, etc.

These approaches lead to some changes in the living pattern of the respondents. Individuals who are already religious-minded become more religious and those who are not religious start believing in God. They keep fasts, attend religious ceremonies like 'Satsang', 'Satvas' (seven days holy discourse delivered by know saints), visit holy shrines, pilgrimage, and even start taking bath on special occasions especially on dark Monday nights.

Astrologers suggest to fast on particular days, for a particular period or time according to the concerned 'stars' of the couple. Suggestions are given based on the horoscope of the couples. Particular gems are also suggested for wearing on fingers. Various modes of *pujas* (worship) are suggested. Religious books are recommended for studying.

Magico-spiritual healers also suggest various ways to cure their childlessness like:

- Taking bath at different places.
- Wearing *jantras* (sacred magical articles).
- Visiting temples for 11 days, 21 days or 40 days.

- Some also suggest regular visits to their place for proper cure.

There are paranoid symptoms also with those who have the problems of infertility. They become a bit sensitive and suspicious. They think that someone is behind their inability to conceive. These people believe in some external forces operating on them. The infertile people find it very difficult to talk to other people about their childlessness because of the lack of self-confidence, and because they have suspicion that their neighbours and relatives mock at them behind their back and abuse them for their inability to conceive. They lack a sense of humour completely (Mathur, 1989).

FIRST MEDICAL CHECK-UP

Hindu marriage has been accepted by the Indian society as a duty to fulfil the religious as well as social objectives. Together with this the second most important objective of marriage is reproduction or childbearing. If the second objective is not fulfilled when the woman cannot conceive, only then the couple recognises the need for medical assistance. But the number of years (of marriage) after which the couple gets their first check-up done depends on a number of points. In the given Table 5.1, the time period of first check-up has been tested on the basis of different variables.

It is clear that rural people are more sensitive and close to the Indian culture and its influence is so heavy on them that their mentality remains rigid. Conclusively, about 40 per cent rural couples and 50 per cent couples living in urban slums get their first check-up done within a year of marriage.

When the period of first check-up was tested on the basis of caste it was observed that most of the Scheduled Tribes (STs) and Other Backward Classes (OBCs) get the check-up done within one year of marriage. Whereas couples belonging to the general category and Scheduled Castes (SCs) are only one-fourth in number; 25 per cent couples belonging to general category got their check-up within one or two years of marriage. The use of contraceptives can be considered as one of the reasons.

Table 5.1

First Check-up

Percentage Distribution of Couples by Selected Background Characteristics

Characteristics	*0-1 Year*	*1-2 Years*	*2-3 Years*	*3-4 Years*	*4+ Years*	*Total Per cent*	*Num-ber*	x^2 *Value/ df and Significance*
Residence								
Rural	38.6	29.5	13.6	11.5	6.8	100.00	88	
Urban slums	48.3	20.7	20.7	10.3	0.0	100.00	29	15.457/8*
Urban	31.7	17.1	25.2	11.4	14.6	100.00	123	
Caste								
General	26.7	25.0	13.3	20.0	15.0	100.00	60	
SC	28.3	25.0	36.7	5.0	5.0	100.00	60	27.599/12**
ST	48.3	18.3	16.7	10.0	6.7	100.00	60	
OBC	41.7	20.0	15.0	10.0	13.3	100.00	60	
Husband's Occupation								
Own business	27.8	17.7	34.3	13.9	6.3	100.00	79	
Service	29.6	26.9	14.8	11.1	17.6	100.00	108	40.977/8**
Agriculture	58.3	20.8	16.7	4.2	0.0	100.00	53	
Total	36.3	22.1	20.4	11.2	10.0	100.00	240	

* Chi-square is significant at the 0.05 level.
** Chi-square is significant at the 0.01 level.

The occupation of the man also affects the first check-up. It is found when out of men belonging to agriculture tasks, 60 per cent get their check-up done within a year of marriage. Out of men holding private jobs more than one-third get their first check-up done between two to three years of marriage. Family planning can be considered as one of the reasons for this.

The time of first check-up was put to the association test (Chi-square) on the basis of various variables. The significant difference between the occupation of man and the first check-up was found to be at .01 level, which makes it clear at the perfect time for childbearing, the knowledge of family planning and the man's occupations are related.

PLACE OF FIRST CHECK-UP (MALE)

Table 5.2 shows the selection of the place of the first medical check-up by childless males, done on the basis of various variables. It is evident that almost half of the male folk living in rural areas get their check-up done in general hospitals. Generally, the rural men find it quite convenient to get checked up in general hospitals. On the contrary, urban men prefer private clinics for the same purpose. More than 40 per cent of the urban men folk get their check-up done in private clinics and only a third of them go to the general hospitals, even though private clinics are costlier than general hospitals.

It is clear that men are hesitant to get their barrenness tested. Quite contrary to this, the type of house also affects the first medical check-up. The men living in *kachcha* houses are not financially sound and cannot afford to go to private clinics. Thus, one out of six males is able to reach out to the private clinics, whereas, every second male is able to get himself tested in general hospitals. Men living in semi-*pucca* houses appeared to be still weaker financially as most of them were comparatively stronger than the rest, financially. Thus, in order to keep their tests a secret and due to their social and economic status, they choose to bear the excessive amount of expenses and get themselves checked-up in private clinics.

When this research was carried out on the basis of caste, it was found that men belonging to scheduled tribe and other backward classes mostly get themselves checked up in general hospitals, whereas, this attitude was not found in men belonging to the general category. When all the various economic groups of men in the general category were combined, it was found that 40 per cent of the men use private clinics and the same percentage of men use the general hospitals. The percentage of men getting their check-up done in health camps, held from time to time, is very less. In the general

Table 5.2
Place of First Check-up (Male)
Percentage Distribution of Men by Selected Background Characteristics

Characteristics	*General Hospital*	*Private Clinic*	*Health Camps*	*No Checking*	*Total Per cent*	*No.*	x^2 *Value/ df and Significance*
Residence							
Rural	52.3	10.2	8.0	29.5	100.00	88	
Urban slums	34.5	17.2	13.8	34.5	100.00	29	35.789/6**
Urban	34.1	41.5	0.8	23.6	100.00	123	
House							
Kachcha	45.7	16.7	6.3	31.3	100.00	48	
Semi-pucca	60.5	8.5	8.5	22.5	100.00	71	37.951/6**
Pucca	27.3	42.1	2.5	28.1	100.00	121	
Caste							
General	40.0	41.7	0.0	18.3	100.00	60	
SC	23.3	21.7	3.3	51.7	100.00	60	43.058/9**
ST	55.0	21.6	11.7	11.7	100.00	60	
OBC	45.0	23.3	5.0	26.7	100.00	60	
Family							
Nuclear	42.0	24.5	7.7	25.8	100.00	143	12.301/3*
Joint	39.2	30.9	1.0	28.9	100.00	97	
Husband's Occupation							
Own business	34.1	38.0	5.1	22.8	100.00	79	
Service	35.2	28.7	0.9	35.2	100.00	108	34.576/6**
Agriculture	62.3	7.5	13.2	17.0	100.00	53	
Wife's Occupation							
Own business	32.0	44.0	0.0	24.0	100.00	25	
Service	21.8	49.1	3.6	25.5	100.00	55	48.530/9**
Agriculture	63.0	18.2	0.6	18.2	100.00	31	
Housewife	50.4	17.8	3.9	27.9	100.00	129	
Monthly Income							
<2000	33.3	8.3	2.8	55.6	100.00	36	
2000-5000	48.3	24.2	7.3	20.2	100.00	124	38.107/9**
5000-8000	31.0	35.6	4.8	28.6	100.00	42	
8000+	20.0	60.0	0.0	20.0	100.00	38	
Total	40.8	27.1	5.0	27.1	100.00	240	

* Chi-square is significant at the 0.05 level.
** Chi-square is significant at the 0.01 level.

category, this percentage becomes zero; the reason may be attributed to the trustworthiness or the doubtful secrecy of these health camps.

The nature of the family of the male respondents has also been considered as one of the important variables and it has been found that men living in nuclear families are more broad or open-minded as compared to men living in joint families. Such men prefer to cut out the extra expenses in private clinics and choose to undergo the check-up in general hospitals.

Figures reveal that only one-fourth of the men living in nuclear families go to private clinics but every third male living in joint family chooses private clinics. The reason for this may be the fear of insult, and also sound economic or financial status, which is comparatively higher in men living in joint families.

Profession of the male also affects the choice of his place of first check-up. Men running their own business possess a different identity in the society. They are quite well known and recognised, therefore about 40 per cent men prefer private clinics to get their tests done. On the other hand, farmers cannot afford to bear such high expenses, thus, two out of every three males get their check-up done in general hospitals.

It is also evident that the choice of first place of male check-up is also affected by the fact whether his wife is a partner in earning money for the family. Men whose wives are working, (every second male) go to private clinics because his social circle is comparatively wider than the rest, also it becomes a must to keep it a secret. On the contrary, if the woman is a housewife or an agricultural worker, the choice of the male is not much affected. About 50.4 per cent and 63 per cent men respectively, unhesitatingly use general hospitals.

In the present age, the monthly income is likely to affect any decision taken by people. As the monthly income of a male increases his inclination towards private clinics also increases. Men earning about Rs. 8,000 do not go to health camps at all, while the percentage of the same increases when we talk about private clinics. Thus, it is clear that a male chooses his place of first medical check-up on the basis of monthly income or economic condition also.

PLACE OF FIRST CHECK-UP (FEMALE)

It is clear that day to day, whether in rural or urban areas, the awareness for medical treatment is getting more evident than before. The common man is more concerned about various health hazards. But, the place of check-up depends on many points, like the expenditure of the check-up, level of education, occupation and income group. One the basis of these points, the choice of the place of first check-up of females in childless couples, was tested.

It is found that more than three-fourths of rural women get their first check-up done in general hospitals, whereas less than 50 per cent of urban women prefer to go to private clinics.

The nature of residence and the kind of house both have an equivalent effect. Among women living in *pucca* houses, every one out of two women prefer to go to private clinics. When the chi-square test was conducted on the nature of residence and the kind of houses, the difference in the significance level was found to be .01 level.

It was also seen that the women falling in the general category do not get checked up on the health camp which are held from time to time; these camps are mostly used by women of the ST category, which is 13 per cent of women. The medical decisions are also affected by occupation. It was found that more than half of the working women chooses private clinics as their first place of check-up, whereas 69 per cent of housewives choose general hospitals. There is a deep association between the place of first check-up and the occupation of women. Chi-square test was conducted and the significance level was found at .01 level. Besides this, family income, husband's occupational condition, nature of family and the effects of thereof have also been shown in Table 5.3.

Table 5.3
Place of First Check-up (Female)
Percentage Distribution of Women by Selected Background Characteristics

Characteristics	*General Hospital*	*Private Clinic*	*Health Camps*	*Total Per cent*	*Number*	*x^2 Value/ df and Significance*
Residence						
Rural	77.3	13.6	9.1	100.00	88	
Urban slums	62.1	24.1	13.8	100.00	29	37.084/4**
Urban	47.4	50.2	2.4	100.00	123	
House						
Kachcha	72.9	18.8	8.3	100.00	48	
Semi-pucca	80.3	11.3	8.4	100.00	71	42.236/4**
Pucca	42.1	53.7	4.2	100.00	121	
Caste						
General	53.3	46.7	0.0	100.00	60	
SC	61.7	31.7	6.6	100.00	60	
ST	63.3	23.3	13.4	100.00	60	14.241/6*
OBC	60.0	35.0	5.0	100.00	60	
Family						
Nuclear	62.9	28.7	8.4	100.00	143	
Joint	54.6	42.3	3.1	100.00	97	6.392/2*
Husband's Occupation						
Own business	43.0	49.4	7.6	100.00	79	
Service	61.1	38.0	0.9	100.00	108	39.690/4**
Agriculture	81.1	3.8	15.1	100.00	53	
Wife's Occupation						
Own business	44.0	56.0	0.0	100.00	25	
Service	38.2	54.5	7.3	100.00	55	
Agriculture	71.0	9.6	19.4	100.00	31	36.657/6**
Housewife	69.0	27.1	3.9	100.00	129	
Monthly Income						
<2000	77.8	19.4	2.8	100.00	36	
2000-5000	61.3	29.0	9.7	100.00	124	
5000-8000	52.3	42.9	4.8	100.00	42	22.324/6**
8000+	53.6	46.4		100.00	38	
Total	59.6	34.2	6.2	100.00	240	

* Chi-square is significant at the 0.05 level.
** Chi-square is significant at the 0.01 level.

DIAGNOSIS FOR INFERTILITY

After the test, out of a total of 240 couples, inability was found in 36 per cent men, whereas among women more than 75 per cent were found unable to conceive. Out of 36 per cent men who were found inable, 6.8 per cent were such who were permanently inable and yet they wanted further tests to be conducted. A minor defect was found only in 15 per cent men. Major defects (but medically curable) were found in 33 men who were hopeful for a child.

After the tests of women, the highest percentage, i.e., more than 35 per cent was found in women whose defects were minor; more than 30 per cent was found with major defects but medically curable and they were temporary. Only about 9 per cent women was declared to be childless because of their defects were not curable.

Table 5.4
Type of Faults

Fault	*Male*		*Female*	
	No.	*Per cent*	*No.*	*Per cent*
Minor	37	15.40	86	35.80
Major but curable	33	13.80	74	30.90
Permanent	16	6.80	21	8.70
NA	154	64.00	59	24.60
Total	240	100.00	240	100.00

PARENTS' REACTION ON SEEING THE REPORT (MALE'S FAULT)

Table 5.5 tries to show the parents' reaction after the report shows that the male is responsible for childlessness. The reactions have been divided and defined into five stages. When the report shows the male's fault, the parents either show sympathy, which is one out of every ten males, or remain neutral which has been found to be for nearly 14 per cent male.

Table 5.5

Reactions of Parents (Male's Fault)

Percentage Distribution of Men by Selected Background Characteristics

Characteristics	*Arguments and Quarrels*	*Tension*	*Avoidance*	*Indifference*	*Sympathy*	*N.A.*	*Total Per cent*	*No.*	*x^2 Value/ df and Significance*
Residence									
Rural	1.1	15.9	2.2	11.4	11.4	58.0	100.00	88	
Urban slums	3.4	0.0	3.4	17.2	20.7	55.3	100.00	29	18.643/10*
Urban	1.6	7.3	0.8	14.6	4.9	70.8	100.00	123	
House									
Kachcha	2.1	6.3	4.2	6.3	12.5	68.6	100.00	48	
Semi-pucca	1.4	16.9	1.4	14.1	16.9	49.3	100.00	71	23.961/10**
Pucca	1.7	6.6	0.8	16.5	3.3	71.1	100.00	121	
Caste									
General	0.0	16.7	1.7	16.7	8.3	56.6	100.00	60	
SC	0.0	3.3	3.3	13.3	1.7	78.4	100.00	60	46.422/15**
ST	3.3	6.7	0.0	11.7	26.7	51.6	100.00	60	
OBC	3.3	11.7	1.7	13.3	0.0	70.0	100.00	60	
Husband's Occupation									
Own business	1.3	12.7	1.3	10.1	2.5	72.1	100.00	79	
Service	1.9	9.3	2.8	15.7	6.5	63.8	100.00	108	24.786/10**
Agriculture	1.9	5.7	0.0	15.1	24.5	52.8	100.00	53	
Wife's Occupation									
Own business	12.0	16.0	8.0	16.0	0.0	48.0	100.00	25	
Service	0.0	1.8	3.6	20.0	3.6	71.0	100.00	55	49.161/15**
Agriculture	0.0	0.0	0.0	9.7	16.1	74.2	100.00	31	
Housewife	0.8	14.0	0.0	11.6	11.6	62.0	100.00	129	
Total	1.7	9.6	1.7	13.8	9.2	64.0	100.00	240	

* Chi-square is significant at the 0.05 level.
** Chi-square is significant at the 0.01 level.

Quarrels and ignorant attitude is very less, i.e., nearly 2 per cent in each category. Not applicable includes the males who did not have any fault in their medical report. The table makes it evident that the percentage of quarrels in rural areas is almost nil (1.1%), but there exists an atmosphere of tension in more than 15 per cent families. Everyone out of 10 families shows sympathy towards the man, whereas in urban men, about 15 per cent of them remain neutral.

The nature of houses and the reactions of parents are also closely associated. Parents of men living in *kachcha* or semi-*pucca* houses show sympathy towards them and this ratio is sometimes greater than 1:8, whereas nearly 17 per cent of men living in *pucca* houses are shown neutrality.

On carrying out the study of reactions on the basis of caste, it came to light that due to childlessness, tensed behaviour towards men is most in the general and OBC category, which is 16.7 per cent and 11.7 per cent respectively, and the same percentage may be used for those who remain neutral.

The occupational background also affects these reactions. Men who are in agricultural occupation are shown sympathy by their parents. This situation has been observed with one-fourth men. Only 5 per cent men had to face arguments and tensions.

The reactions were observed on the basis of the nature of marriage, kind of family and the occupation of the woman and no significant difference was found. It was found at 0.1 level in the occupational situations, caste and the nature of residence of men and women.

PARENTS' REACTION ON SEEING THE REPORT (FEMALE'S FAULT)

An Indian woman should be an ideal wife, an ideal daughter-in-law and an ideal mother. She lives her life on this principle. Reactions of the mother-in-law and father-in-law, when their daughter-in-law is not able to give them an heir to their family and fulfil their dreams and aspirations are shown in

Table 5.6 It shows that the women face a tensed atmosphere when the report shows their fault, whereas quarrels and fights crop up in about nearly 23 per cent houses. Only 5 per cent parents remain neutral. Not applicable includes the females who did not have any fault in their medical report.

Table 5.6

Reactions of Parents (Female's Fault)
Percentage Distribution of Women by Selected Background Characteristics

Characteristics	*Arguments and Quarrels*	*Tension*	*Avoidance*	*Indifference*	*Sympathy*	*N.A.*	*Total Per cent*	*No.*	*x^2 Value/ df and Significance*
Residence									
Rural	14.80	35.20	5.70	5.70	8.00	30.60	100.00	88	
Urban slums	48.30	17.20	17.20	0.00	0.00	17.30	100.00	29	23.184/10**
Urban	22.00	30.90	9.80	6.50	8.90	21.90	100.00	123	
Caste									
General	16.70	11.70	3.30	11.70	25.00	31.60	100.00	60	
SC	35.00	28.30	18.30	6.70	0.00	11.70	100.00	60	72.304/15**
ST	20.00	40.00	8.30	1.70	1.70	28.30	100.00	60	
OBC	18.30	43.30	6.70	1.70	3.30	26.70	100.00	60	
Husband's Occupation									
Own business	17.70	35.40	10.10	2.50	3.80	30.50	100.00	79	
Service	21.30	23.10	10.20	8.30	13.00	24.10	100.00	108	21.364/10**
Agriculture	32.10	39.60	5.70	3.80	1.90	16.90	100.00	53	
Wife's Occupation									
Own business	28.00	0.00	12.00	8.00	8.00	44.00	100.00	25	
Service	18.20	32.70	18.20	7.30	7.30	16.30	100.00	55	31.040/15**
Agriculture	35.50	35.50	9.70	6.50	3.20	9.60	100.00	31	
Housewife	20.20	34.90	4.70	3.90	8.50	27.80	100.00	129	
Total	22.50	30.80	9.20	5.40	7.50	24.60	100.00	240	

* Chi-square is significant at the 0.05 level.
** Chi-square is significant at the 0.01 level.

The given table makes it quite evident that argument and quarrels are three times greater in urban slums than in rural areas. In rural families more than 35 per cent women have to face tensions in the family. The situation of urban women is more or less the same. The reactions of parents were tested on the basis of caste and it was found that the arguments and quarrels are most in SCs and STs. Nearly 35 per cent families of SCs and one out of every 5 families in STs have quarrels. Also in 40 per cent families of STs, childless women were given a tensed environment.

The occupation of a woman also affects the reaction of her family. It has been observed that service class women do not have to suffer arguments and quarrels but about one-third of them have to undergo tension. The reactions of parents were also studied on the basis of the nature of marriage and the kind of family. On conducting the significance test, on the basis of the occupation of a woman, the nature of residence and caste, significant differences were found in the reactions.

REACTION OF RELATIVES WHEN CHILDLESSNESS IS DUE TO MALE

Table 5.7 shows that when the man is responsible for childlessness the relatives are not much affected by it. Their reactions are strong when the woman is responsible. The couples whose relatives remain neutral are greatest in number. In the case of man, family arguments and quarrels are very less. In the villages, only 1 per cent couples and in the slums 3.4 per cent couples have had to face conflicts or struggles. Most of the couples' relative remained dumb or neutral in this context. One out of every ten couples living in nuclear families had to face tension.

Table 5.7

Reactions of Relatives (Male's Fault)

Percentage Distribution of Men by Selected Background Characteristics

Characteristics	*Arguments and Quarrels*	*Tension*	*Avoidance*	*Indifference*	*Sympathy*	*N.A.*	*Total Per cent*	*No.*	*x^2 Value/ df and Significance*
Residence									
Rural	1.10	17.00	5.70	17.00	1.10	58.10	100.00	88	
Urban slums	3.40	3.40	13.80	20.70	3.40	55.30	100.00	29	22.017/10**
Urban	0.00	6.50	1.60	17.10	4.10	70.70	100.00	123	
House									
Kachcha	2.10	8.30	8.30	8.30	4.20	68.80	100.00	48	
Semi-pucca	1.40	21.10	5.60	19.70	2.80	49.40	100.00	71	24.816/10**
Pucca	0.00	4.10	2.50	19.80	2.80	70.80	100.00	121	
Family									
Nuclear	0.70	11.90	7.70	20.30	3.50	55.90	100.00	60	14.497/5*
Joint	1.00	7.20	0.00	13.40	2.10	76.30	100.00	60	
Total	0.80	10.00	4.80	17.50	2.90	64.00	100.00	240	

* Chi-square is significant at the 0.05 level.

** Chi-square is significant at the 0.01 level.

REACTIONS OF RELATIVES WHEN CHILDLESSNESS IS DUE TO FEMALE

Table 5.8 shows the reaction of relatives and family, after the first medical check-up shows that the woman is responsible for childlessness. The reactions have been divided into five levels, out of which two have been taken as extreme arguments and quarrels and sympathy. These reactions have been tested on the basis of various variables. Not applicable includes the males who did not have any fault in their medical report.

The fact is that nearly 31 per cent women said that they had to face tension from their relatives, and a total of 18 per cent women had to face arguments and quarrels also. The least percentage is of these women who gain sympathy; their percentage amount to 8 per cent.

Table 5.8
Reactions of Relatives (Female's Fault)
Percentage Distribution of Women by Selected Background Characteristics

Characteristics	*Arguments and Quarrels*	*Tension*	*Avoidance*	*Indifference*	*Sympathy*	*N.A.*	*Total Per cent*	*No.*	x^2 *Value/ df and Significance*
Residence									
Rural	12.50	33.00	8.00	8.00	8.00	30.50	100	88	
Urban slums	37.90	27.60	17.20	0.00	0.00	17.30	100	29	18.831/10*
Urban	17.10	30.10	9.80	11.40	9.80	21.80	100	123	
Caste									
General	13.30	13.30	3.30	13.30	25.00	31.80	100	60	
SC	23.30	40.00	18.30	6.70	0.00	11.70	100	60	57.190/15**
ST	20.00	33.30	11.70	5.00	1.70	28.30	100	60	
OBC	15.00	36.70	6.70	10.00	5.00	26.60	100	60	
Wife's Occupation									
Own business	12.00	8.00	12.00	16.00	8.00	44.00	100	25	
Service	18.20	25.50	18.20	10.90	10.90	16.30	100	55	27.798/15*
Agriculture	29.00	41.90	9.70	6.50	3.20	9.70	100	31	
Housewife	16.30	34.90	6.20	7.00	7.80	27.80	100	129	
Type of Marriage									
Love marriage	15.20	12.10	18.20	12.10	0.00	42.40	100	33	15.549/5**
Arranged marriage	18.40	33.80	8.70	8.20	9.20	21.70	100	207	
Total	17.90	30.80	10.00	8.80	7.90	24.60	100	240	

* Chi-square is significant at the 0.05 level.
** Chi-square is significant at the 0.01 level.

In urban slums, nearly 38 per cent women have to face quarrels and fights in their families while the percentage of women gaining sympathy is zero; this makes it quite clear that the nature of residence affects the human behaviour. On the contrary, in cities, it has been observed that couples do not quarrel openly but develop a mental tension between each other. One out of every three couples has to face such a tension.

When the study of reactions was made on the basis of caste it was found that families belonging to the general category show a sympathetic behaviour. It also revealed that 25 per cent of women who were found to be responsible for childlessness did not have to face a tense atmosphere or neglected behaviour. On the contrary, about one-third of women belonging to the Scheduled Caste, Scheduled Tribe and Other Backward Class category faced a tense behaviour in their family.

The occupational status of women has also been considered as an important variable and the conclusion drawn from the study thus made is that women who are in the agricultural field have to suffer a lot of struggles, quarrels and arguments in their family. The percentage of such women is 29, together with 40 per cent women who have to undergo mental tension.

Love marriages have not yet been given a respectable recognition and position in the Indian society. Therefore, when a woman is found barren (after love marriage) she does not get any sympathy and about 20 per cent women have had to feel the pinch of being ignored or neglected.

When the significance of reactions of relatives towards the report was tested by the chi-square test, then .01 level difference was found on the basis of caste and marriage. Whereas, the significance was found to be .05 level in the context of the nature of residence and the tenure of marriage. Thus, it is evident that the nature of residence widely affects the attitude of people. The association was also studied on the kind of family, kind of marriage, but no significant difference was found.

REACTIONS OF CO-WORKERS AT THE WORKPLACE (MALE'S FAULT)

Since in today's busy world people are engrossed in solving their own problems and meeting their own needs and do not bother about the other person's troubles, the report of childlessness of a man did not have much impact on his co-workers.

Table 5.9 shows the reactions of co-workers at the workplace when they come to know about childlessness.

Table 5.9

Reactions of Co-workers (Male's Fault)

Percentage Distribution of Men by Selected Background Characteristics

Characteristics	*Avoi-dance*	*Neutral*	*Sym-pathy*	*N.A.*	*Total Per cent*	*Number*	x^2 *Value/ df and Significance*
Residence							
Rural	2.30	39.80	0.00	57.90	100.00	88	
Urban slums	0.00	37.90	6.90	55.20	100.00	29	13.947/6*
Urban	1.60	26.80	0.90	70.70	100.00	123	
House							
Kachcha	0.00	31.30	0.00	68.70	100.00	48	
Semi-pucca	2.80	45.10	2.80	49.30	100.00	71	11.801/6*
Pucca	1.70	26.40	0.80	71.10	100.00	121	
Caste							
General	1.70	38.30	3.30	56.70	100.00	60	
SC	0.00	21.70	0.00	78.30	100.00	60	16.064/9*
ST	1.70	45.00	1.70	51.60	100.00	60	
OBC	3.30	26.70	0.00	70.00	100.00	60	
Total	1.70	32.90	1.40	64.00	100.00	240	

* Chi-square is significant at the 0.05 level.
** Chi-square is significant at the 0.01 level.

Especially in rural areas, only 2 per cent men are looked down upon, whereas men generally do not experience this kind of state at all. Most co-workers remain indifferent or neutral to this state. The association was also studied on the kind of family, kind of marriage, but no significant difference was found.

REACTIONS OF CO-WORKERS AT THE WORKPLACE (FEMALE'S FAULT)

Table 5.10 shows the mixed reactions of co-workers when the woman is responsible for childlessness. When the reaction was studied on the basis of the residence, it was found that the co-workers living in cities showed sympathy towards women. The percentage of co-workers living in cities works out to 13 per cent whereas one-fourth co-workers dwelling in urban slums show sympathy.

Table 5.10

Reactions of Co-workers (Female's Fault)
Percentage Distribution of Women by Selected Background Characteristics

Characteristics	*Avoidance*	*Neutral*	*Sympathy*	*N.A.*	*Total Per cent*	*Number*	*x^2 Value/ df and Significance*
Residence							
Rural	0.00	14.80	2.20	83.00	100.00	88	
Urban slums	0.00	27.60	24.10	48.30	100.00	29	18.145/4**
Urban	0.00	21.10	13.00	65.90	100.00	123	
Caste							
General	0.00	20.00	1.70	78.30	100.00	60	
SC	0.00	30.00	20.00	50.00	100.00	60	19.829/6**
ST	0.00	15.00	8.30	76.70	100.00	60	
OBC	0.00	13.30	11.70	75.00	100.00	60	
Wife's Occupation							
Own business	0.00	16.00	4.00	80.00	100.00	25	
Service	0.00	43.60	38.20	18.20	100.00	55	161.803/6**
Agriculture	0.00	58.10	9.70	32.30	100.10	31	
Housewife	0.00	0.00	0.00	100.00	100.00	129	
Total	0.00	19.60	10.40	70.00	100.00	240	

* Chi-square is significant at the 0.05 level.
** Chi-square is significant at the 0.01 level.

Not applicable includes the women who are either housewives or did not have any fault. When the study was carried out on the basis of caste, it was observed that working women are either shown sympathy by their co-workers or they remain indifferent or neutral. None of them was getting avoidance.

Business has also affected the reactions of the co-workers. More than 38 per cent of service class women have been shown sympathy. The reason for this vast difference in reactions may be attributed to the fact that the social circle of the service class women is comparatively larger than the women working in agricultural fields.

CHANGE IN EATING HABITS ALONG WITH MEDICAL TREATMENT

As this study is clinic based, it has been found that almost all men who comprise of 36 per cent of couples did take treatment. When they were asked about the control and change of eating habits based on the medical treatment and experience, it was found that one out of ten men changed eating habits according to the medical treatment or on what he was advised (Table 5.11). Due to the family pressure, religious sentiments, self-beliefs, women are more prone to change their eating habits. As many as 25 per cent women stopped the intake of various food items and took to the eating habits suggested by the family members.

Table 5.11

Change in Eating Habits Along With the Medical Treatment

Change	*Male*		*Female*	
	Number	*Percentage*	*Number*	*Percentage*
Left egg and non-veg	13	5.40	10	4.20
Left cold/hot eatables	10	4.20	25	10.40
Left food made in market	0	0.00	25	10.40
No change	217	90.40	180	75.00
Total	240	100.00	240	100.00

When asked in detail, it was revealed that due to some religious reasons men stopped taking alcohol and non-vegetarian food and out of these 10 per cent of the men forsake egg and non-vegetarian food and nearly 4 per cent men stopped the intake of cooling foods like curd, cumin seeds, etc. They say that according to the family members, cold foodstuffs have a negative impact on fertility. So they forsake such foodstuffs for the satisfaction of the family members.

Out of the three-fourths women taking treatment, one-fourth of them have been known to have brought a change in their eating habits. Out of them, the percentage of women forsaking egg and non-vegetarian was the lowest; only about 4 per cent women forsook these foodstuffs. Out of these one-fourth women, the percentage of women eating non-vegetarian foods was also less. But on the other hand, the percentage of women who forsook the intake of junk food was nearly 10 per cent. The junk food or market food includes food made in market and food made in other's houses (except in relatives' house). On the advice of family members, nearly 10 per cent stopped the intake of cold, hot and oily foodstuffs; especially the women who had an abortion did not eat jaggery, spices, curd, oily food stuffs as well as cold food stuffs. In this way, the effect of home remedies together with medical treatment was seen on women.

KINDS OF ALTERNATIVE THERAPIES (MALE)

Table 5.12 shows the various alternatives other than the medical treatment by the male and these have been tested on the basis of various variables. The significance test has also been performed at .01 level and .05 level by chi-square.

In the use of alternative therapies, 12.1 per cent men believe in *puja* or worship, whereas less than 1 per cent men go for witchcraft. Among STs, 23.3 per cent men use witchcraft and the like remedies. A deep association has been noticed between the kind of houses and the choice of treatment. Around 15.5 per cent men living in semi-*pucca* houses believe in witchcraft and about one-third men also conduct *pujas* and various other rituals along with witchcraft. Whereas, people living in *pucca* houses do not believe in witchcraft, 13 per cent

Table 5.12

Kinds of Alternative Therapies (Male)

Percentage Distribution of men by Selected Background Characteristics

Characteristics	Spiritual Healing	Witchcraft	Witchcraft & Spiritual Healing	Wish Making	Witchcraft, Spiritual Healing & Wish Making	Worship	Wish Making & Worship	Witch-craft, Wish Making & Worship	Witch-craft, Spiritual Healing, Wish-making & Worship	Number	x^2 Value/ df and Significance
House											
Kachcha	0.00	2.10	2.10	14.60	16.70	8.30	8.30	0.00	33.30	48	
Semi-pucca	1.40	0.00	15.50	8.50	9.90	7.00	2.80	2.80	31.00	71	37.459/18**
Pucca	5.00	0.00	5.80	13.20	6.60	9.10	5.00	0.00	19.80	121	
Duration of Marriage											
>3	0.00	0.00	0.00	0.00	0.00	0.00	50.00	0.00	50.00	4	
3-8	1.00	0.00	2.10	9.30	11.80	10.30	4.10	0.00	20.60	97	88.885/36**
8-13	7.40	0.00	16.20	17.60	11.80	5.90	4.40	0.00	19.10	68	
13+	2.50	3.20	17.20	22.20	12.90	17.90	9.00	6.50	8.60	31	

Contd...

Contd...

Caste											
General	0.00	0.00	0.00	5.00	1.70	1.70	10.00	0.00	35.00	60	
SC	0.00	0.00	3.30	20.00	23.30	15.00	6.70	0.00	8.30	60	
ST	3.30	1.70	23.30	15.00	5.00	1.70	0.00	0.00	33.30	60	109.185/27**
OBC	8.30	0.00	5.00	8.30	8.30	15.00	3.30	3.30	26.70	60	
Family											
Nuclear	2.10	0.00	9.80	13.30	13.30	9.80	1.40	0.00	25.20	143	
Joint	4.10	1.00	5.20	10.30	4.10	6.20	10.30	2.10	26.85	97	22.907/9**
Total	2.90	0.40	7.90	12.10	9.60	8.30	5.00	0.80	25.80	240	

* Chi-square is significant at the 0.05 level.
** Chi-square is significant at the 0.01 level.

men make wishes in temples or at any holy place. It is the men living in *kachcha* houses who have a strong belief in the use of other alternatives. One-third men use other alternatives except witchcraft. The significant difference in chi-square test is found to be at .01 level, which makes it clear that there is a huge difference in these alternatives on the basis of the residence.

The period of marriage also affects the use of alternatives. Except *puja* (worship) and making wishes, no other alternatives have been used within the first three years of marriage and 50 per cent men too only did this. But between three to eight years of marriage these alternatives get the attention of many men and one out of 10 men starts offering prayers and worship. Between the married life of 8 and 13 years men start getting attracted towards nearly all the alternatives and start performing rituals, offering prayers, pledging vows and also take to witchcraft.

Caste and practice of alternative are also deeply linked to each other. The use of witchcraft is greater among the STs. One-third men perform this, whereas OBCs lay more stress on offering prayers and worship. Among other backward classes, 15 per cent men perform puja. The nature of family was also considered as an important variable and the conducted studies reveal that men belonging to nuclear families mostly make wishes; they amount to 13 per cent. Whereas men belonging to joint families believe in witchcraft.

KINDS OF ALTERNATIVE THERAPIES (FEMALE)

With the help of various government organisations and NGOs, allopathy has spread to most of the villages, and with the help of health camps, satellite hospitals, primary health centres, etc., the people have been educated about all the latest diseases, their symptoms and their cures. Yet, their faith in alternative therapy is not shaken.

More than 80 per cent women are embracing other alternatives together with medical treatment (Table 5.13). On

Table 5.13

Kinds of Alternative Therapies (Female)

Percentage Distribution of Women by Selected Background Characteristics

Characteristics	*Spiritual Healing*	*Witch-craft*	*Witch-craft & Spiritual Healing*	*Wish Making*	*Witch-craft, Spiritual Healing & Wish Making*	*Worship*	*Wish Making & Worship*	*Witch-craft, Wish Making & Worship*	*Witch-craft, Spiritual Healing, Wish Making & Worship*	*Number*	*x^2 Value/ df and Significance*
Residence											
Rural	2.30	1.10	9.10	6.80	14.80	8.00	0.00	0.00	40.90	88	
Urban slums	0.00	0.00	10.30	17.20	20.70	10.30	3.40	0.00	34.50	29	28.170/18*
Urban	2.40	0.00	2.40	12.20	15.40	5.70	8.90	1.60	31.70	123	
House											
Kachcha	0.00	0.00	8.30	8.30	18.80	4.20	0.00	0.00	45.80	48	
Semi-pucca	0.00	1.40	8.50	9.90	18.30	4.20	2.80	2.80	42.30	71	33.273/18**
Pucca	4.10	0.00	3.30	12.40	13.20	6.60	8.30	0.00	27.30	121	
Duration of Marriage											
>3	0.00	0.00	0.00	0.00	0.00	25.00	0.00	0.00	75.00	4	
3-8	0.00	0.00	5.20	10.30	18.60	6.20	8.20	0.00	28.90	97	
8-13	4.4	1.5	5.9	13.2	16.20	0.00	2.90	0.00	36.80	68	51.759/36*
13-18	6.50	0.00	3.20	9.70	19.40	12.90	3.20	6.50	29.00	31	
18+	0.00	0.00	10.00	10.00	7.50	5.00	2.50	0.00	50.00	40	

Contd...

Contd...

Caste											
General	0.00	0.00	0.00	5.00	8.30	1.70	10.00	0.00	41.70	60	
SC	3.30	1.70	8.30	13.30	26.70	6.70	5.00	0.00	23.30	60	55.807/27**
ST	1.70	0.00	10.00	13.30	15.00	1.70	1.70	0.00	46.70	60	
OBC	3.30	0.00	5.00	11.70	13.30	11.70	3.30	3.30	30.00	60	
Husband's Occupation											
Own business	2.50	0.00	1.30	12.70	15.20	7.60	3.80	2.50	34.20	79	
Service	0.90	0.00	5.60	13.00	12.00	4.60	8.30	0.00	32.40	108	33.278/18**
Agriculture	3.80	0.90	13.20	3.80	24.50	3.80	0.00	0.00	43.40	53	
Wife's Occupation											
Own business	0.00	0.00	0.00	4.00	16.00	16.00	12.00	0.00	40.00	25	
Service	3.60	0.00	1.80	7.30	9.10	5.50	7.30	0.00	23.60	55	52.307/27**
Agriculture	0.00	0.00	16.10	3.20	22.60	6.50	0.00	0.00	45.20	31	
Housewife	2.30	0.80	6.20	7.00	17.10	3.10	3.90	1.60	37.20	129	
Total	2.10	0.40	5.80	10.80	15.80	5.40	5.00	0.80	35.40	240	

* Chi-square is significant at the 0.05 level.

** Chi-square is significant at the 0.01 level.

conducting the study on the basis of the native of residence, it was found that about 40 per cent of women living in rural areas opt for magico-spiritual witchcraft, rituals and worship. In this case, the percentage of worship is 8 per cent only.

On the whole, no change has been found in the attitude of the urban women; but around one-third of them opt for witchcraft, magico-spiritual methods, wish making, worshipping, etc. At the same time, it is note worthy that none of the urban woman trusts only witchcraft.

Studies were also conducted on the type of house and it was seen that 45 per cent of women living in *kachcha* and semi-*pucca* houses embrace all the alternative measures, whereas only one-fourth women living in *pucca* houses believe in them.

The effect of period of marriage on the use of alternative measures was also studied. The results showed significant difference at .05 level. Among the couples who have completed three years of marriage, out of them 75 per cent women embrace alternative measures. And out of those who have completed over eighteen years of marriage, 50 per cent women support witchcraft, magico-spiritual and wish making. It is a surprising fact that in the collected data a vast difference has been found on the basis of caste. The percentage of women using alternative measure in the general and scheduled tribes is 42 per cent and 47 per cent respectively. Whereas 23 per cent women of SCs and 30 per cent women of other backward classes believe in them.

The occupation of the wife also affects the attitude of the couple. Through the study, the percentage of working women believing on alternative measures was found to be only 23 per cent. These women consider the alternative therapies as superstition. This kind of belief may be attributed to the open-mindedness and the modernised thinking, gained through contact with the external world.

The occupation of the wife and use of alternative therapies was put to chi-square and the significant difference was found at .01 level.

With respect to the use of alternative therapies, the behaviour of men has been found to differ with respect to that of women. Nearly 20 per cent of women living in slums go for witchcraft and wish making. The nature of family was also studied but no significant different was found.

USE OF SCIENTIFIC AND MODERN MEANS FOR OBTAINING A CHILD

Table 5.14 shows the opinion of couples on the use of scientific and modern means for obtaining a child and also it has been made clear how these opinions affect various variables. In the present age, on one hand, moral and social standards are being avoided and things like surrogate motherhood are being given recognition. On the other hand, there are people who hesitate to use scientific means and prefer to fast and perform many other rituals to obtain a child. They believe that a child should only be born naturally. The study was made on the basis of the women's age and it was observed that most women above 40 years of age do not agree to use any scientific method of treatment; only 11 per cent agree to it. The age of men also affects this decision. Around 63 per cent of men between the age of 35-39 years were prepared to use the scientific methods.

Even after three years of marriage, childless couples are double-minded on whether to have a child naturally or to use some scientific method. But 60 per cent of couples who remain childless even after 13 years of marriage, are prepared to use modern methods of having a child. When the study was made on the basis of caste, it was observed that SCs and OBCs are more broad-minded and affirm the use of modern means of having a child. But it is also true that they do not want to forgo the traditional means as well. Therefore, two-thirds of SCs and more than half of the other backward classes support traditional means.

It is a fact that using modern as well as scientific means is quite an expensive decision and it is difficult to decide whether this decision will be supported or not. On studying the table, it will be evident that those whose family income is above Rs. 8,000 support this decision.

Table 5.14

Use of Scientific and Modern Means for Obtaining a Child
Percentage Distribution of Couples by Selected Background Characteristics

Characteristics	*Yes*	*No*	*Total Per cent*	*Number*
Current Age				
19-24	51.90	48.10	100.00	54
25-29	62.70	37.30	100.00	83
30-34	51.00	49.00	100.00	51
35-39	66.70	33.30	100.00	18
40+	11.80	88.20	100.00	34
Husband's Age				
19-24	50.00	50.00	100.00	6
25-29	54.40	45.60	100.00	57
30-34	58.70	41.30	100.00	75
35-39	63.20	36.80	100.00	57
40+	17.80	82.20	100.00	45
Duration of Marriage				
<3	50.00	50.00	100.00	4
3-8	59.80	40.20	100.00	97
8-13	51.50	48.50	100.00	68
13-18	61.30	38.70	100.00	31
18+	20.00	80.00	100.00	40
Caste				
General	43.30	56.70	100.00	60
SC	65.00	35.00	100.00	60
ST	40.00	60.00	100.00	60
OBC	55.00	45.00	100.00	60
Monthly Income				
<2000	41.70	58.30	100.00	36
2000-5000	52.40	47.60	100.00	124
5000-8000	47.60	52.40	100.00	42
8000+	57.90	42.10	100.00	38
Total	50.80	49.20	100.00	240

MODERN MEANS FOR OBTAINING A CHILD

Table 5.15 shows the data collected from couples who have used the modern and scientific means to produce a child and they were questioned about the kind of scientific and modern methods used. Many factors affect the choice of methods. Not applicable is used for almost half of the couples who do not want to use the scientific and modern methods. Out of the remaining 50.8 per cent couples, less than 10 per cent couples seem to be prepared for test-tube babies. Men between the age of 19-24 years want to embrace other means expect test-tube babies, as long as this remains a legal means. More than one-third couples having a love marriage are eager to have a child by any possible means. The above-mentioned methods were also studied with respect to the nature of residence, type of house, husband's and wife's occupation but no significant difference has been known.

As the age of men and women advances, they become keen to have a child anyhow. But one-third of women between the age group of 25-29, believe that the procedure should be a recognised one, while one-fourth of men in the same age group are ready to use any method as long as it can get them child. When asked about test-tube babies, 15 per cent women in the age group of 25-29 years were in affirmation.

When questioned about the replacement of man or woman for a fixed tenure, nearly all the couples said that this kind of practise is only possible in the western countries and will be considered as a sin in the Indian society. Within three years of marriage 50 per cent childless couples are ready to undergo any recognised treatment but do not give their consent for test-tube babies. It has also been observed that after 8-13 years of marriage, one out of every eight couples give their affirmation for this solution as well. Knowing that to have a test-tube baby is very expensive, and cannot be afforded/borne by every couple, only 16 per cent of couples, who have a monthly income of more than Rs. 8,000, give their consent towards it.

Table 5.15

Modern Methods to Produce a Child
Percentage Distribution of Couples by Selected Background Characteristics

Characteristics	*Test-Tube Baby*	*Other Reco-gnised Methods*	*Any*	*N.A.*	*Total Per cent*	*No.*	x^2 *Value/ df and Significance*
Current Age							
19-24	3.70	24.10	24.10	48.10	100.00	54	
25-29	15.70	34.90	12.00	37.40	100.00	83	
30-34	9.60	13.70	27.70	49.00	100.00	51	42.382/12**
35-39	11.10	33.30	22.30	33.30	100.00	18	
40+	2.90	5.90	2.90	88.30	100.00	34	
Husband's Age							
19-24	0.00	50.00	0.00	50.00	100.00	6	
25-29	8.80	22.80	22.80	45.60	100.00	57	
30-34	18.70	25.30	14.70	41.30	100.00	75	40.787/12**
35-39	3.50	33.50	26.50	36.50	100.00	57	
40+	4.40	6.70	6.70	82.20	100.00	45	
Duration of Marriage							
<3	0.00	50.00	0.00	50.00	100.00	4	
3-8	10.30	26.80	22.70	40.20	100.00	97	
8-13	13.20	20.60	17.60	48.60	100.00	68	24.808/12**
13-18	9.70	35.50	16.10	38.70	100.00	31	
18+	2.50	10.00	7.50	80.00	100.00	40	
Caste							
General	8.30	13.30	21.70	56.70	100.00	60	
SC	13.30	25.00	26.70	35.00	100.00	60	18.320/9*
ST	5.00	25.00	10.00	60.00	100.00	60	
OBC	11.70	31.70	11.60	45.00	100.00	60	
Family							
Nuclear	6.30	23.10	19.60	51.00	100.00	143	14.821/3*
Joint	14.40	24.70	14.50	46.40	100.00	97	
Monthly Income							
<2000	13.90	22.20	5.60	58.30	100.00	36	
2000-5000	7.30	24.20	21.00	47.50	100.00	124	22.666/9*
5000-8000	7.10	23.60	16.70	52.60	100.00	42	
8000+	15.80	23.70	18.40	42.10	100.00	38	
Type of Marriage							
Love marriage	9.10	12.10	36.40	42.40	100.00	33	
Arranged marriage	9.70	25.60	14.50	50.20	100.00	207	10.322/3**
Total	9.60	23.80	17.50	49.10	100.00	240	

* Chi-square is significant at the 0.05 level.
** Chi-sSquare is significant at the 0.01 level.

Many couples including those who had love marriage are generally perturbed due to childlessness and so more than a third of such couples are ready to use any means. But couples, who had arranged marriages, would decide whether to undergo recognised treatments or for test-tube babies.

Any scientific or modern means is considered as a method, which is not necessarily accepted by family or society but can give a child. During this study, many incidences were found to explore the secrets which are more likely unethical in Indian society. Doctors themselves told that they do it with their patient's consent and childless couples also agreed upon this that they are confident about their confidentiality. The childless couples need a child so badly that they agree to do anything unethical - even sexual relationship with other persons.

Type of residence, kind of house, caste and type of family were also taken as the basis of study of the choice of solutions by the couples.

REASONS FOR NOT USING MODERN MEANS

The status of women in the Indian society is supreme. The dignity or honour of a woman is linked with her family, society and the country as a whole. Padmini's 'Jauhar' is an ideal example. That is, an Indian woman can be likened to Pannadhay who sacrificed her only son for her country, and she would not break the moral values and ethics of her country to fulfil her selfish motives and desires. This is the reason why many couples consider the use of scientific and modern means as against their social values. On being questioned about the reasons for not using the new scientific and modern methods of childbearing, most childless couples (43.3%) accepted that child should be conceived in a natural way. One-fourth of them stated that their values do not allow them to tamper with nature.

As many as 85 per cent women above the age of 40 years and 56 per cent couples belonging to the general category, consider the natural way of childbearing as the only appropriate way.

This is especially true for the couples in villages who believe that a child is a gift of God. Almost 42 per cent couples take childlessness as a normal state. And, about one-fourth of childless couples hesitate to undergo a treatment for fear of family, kinship, and some for fear of society.

Table 5.16

Reasons for Not Using Scientific and Modern Means
Percentage Distribution of Couples by Selected Background Characteristics

Characteristics	*Values Don't Allow*	*By the Natural Way*	*Fear of Family*	*Fear of Society*	*Number*
Residence	**				
Rural	30.70	42.00	25.00	28.40	88
Urban slums	3.40	48.30	27.60	20.70	29
Urban	22.00	43.10	17.10	17.90	123
Current Age	**	**	**	**	
19-24	31.50	46.30	18.50	24.10	54
25-29	19.30	28.90	20.50	18.10	83
30-34	13.70	43.10	23.50	23.50	51
35-39	0.00	22.20	0.00	0.00	18
40+	44.10	85.30	35.30	38.20	34
Husband's Age	**	**			
19-24	50.00	50.00	16.70	16.70	6
25-29	29.80	40.40	19.30	24.60	57
30-34	13.30	32.00	20.00	17.30	75
35-39	14.00	33.30	17.50	17.50	57
40+	37.80	77.80	31.10	33.30	45
Duration of Marriage	**	**	*		
<3	0.00	50.00	0.00	0.00	4
3-8	24.70	39.20	16.50	18.60	97
8-13	23.50	38.20	29.40	27.90	68
13-18	0.00	22.60	9.70	9.70	31
18+	37.50	77.50	30.00	32.50	40

Contd...

Contd...

Caste				*	
General	33.30	56.70	23.30	33.30	60
SC	15.00	31.70	21.70	21.70	60
ST	21.70	43.30	21.70	23.30	60
OBC	21.70	41.70	18.30	10.00	60
Family					
Nuclear	21.00	42.00	21.70	21.70	143
Joint	25.80	45.40	20.60	22.70	97
Wife's Occupation	*				
Own business	8.00	40.00	16.00	16.00	25
Service	14.50	38.20	21.80	18.20	55
Agriculture	29.00	61.30	29.00	29.00	31
Housewife	27.90	41.90	20.20	23.30	129
Monthly Income		*			
<2000	25.00	44.40	27.80	27.80	36
2000-5000	22.60	42.70	25.00	23.40	124
5000-8000	28.60	47.60	16.70	23.80	42
8000+	15.80	39.50	7.90	10.50	38
Type of Marriage			*	*	
Love marriage	21.20	33.30	9.10	12.10	33
Arranged marriage	23.20	44.90	23.20	23.70	207
Total	22.90	43.30	21.30	22.10	240

* Chi-square is significant at the 0.05 level.
** Chi-square is significant at the 0.01 level.

When this hesitation is studied in context with age, it is seen that women between the age group of 30-34 years do not want to get treated by using scientific and modern means for childlessness. This percentage increases to 85 per cent in the women of age above 40 years. Thus, it is evident that with age the consciousness or fear of the family and society also increases and women concentrate only on children who are naturally born.

It has been observed that one-third men above the age of 40 years fear the society. Thus, more than three-fourths of the male population refuse to undergo treatment for childlessness.

Couples, who are married for 13 to 18 years, do not bother about values or society and openly advocate the use of the modern means.

The opinions or views of couples were also studied on the basis of the nature of residence, type of house, husband's and wife's occupation and the kind of marriage, but no significant difference was found.

REACTIONS OF PARENTS, RELATIVES AND CO-WORKERS ON FIRST MEDICAL REPORT OF CHILDLESSNESS

Reactions of parents, relatives and co-workers were studied (Table 5.17) when they got the first medical report of childlessness. It was found that where males were found responsible for childlessness, gender bias was seen in every category. Respondents from all the three settings agreed that couples especially females had to face more quarrels and avoidance by their in-laws. Parents of the couples, residing either in *kachcha* house or in *pucca* house, often made the females realise that the family was lacking a child because of her. The females also had to face the negative reactions in the wider society, i.e., relatives and co-workers as people expected childbirth soon after marriage. In majority of cases, parents and relatives were found sympathetic towards the male after getting the report, but they passed comments to hurt the females. No significant difference was found in the reactions of parents and relatives on the basis of duration of marriage.

Most of the co-workers of males in rural settings remained indifferent, as they wanted to avoid the discussion about the male's fault. In the urban slums, co-workers of female respondents avoided their company after knowing about their sterility.

Couples engaged in agriculture found it difficult to reveal about their medical confirmation to their parents, as they were afraid of serious consequences. It was found that females relating to farming occupation had faced more quarrels and

Table 5.17

Reactions of Parents, Relatives and Co-workers on First Medical Report of Childlessness
Percentage Distribution of Couples by Selected Background Characteristics

Characteristics	*Parent's Quarrels and Avoidance*		*Relative's Quarrels and Avoidance*		*Co-worker's Avoidance*		*No.*
	Male's Fault	*Female's Fault*	*Male's Fault*	*Female's Fault*	*Male's Fault*	*Female's Fault*	
Residence	*	**		*		**	
Rural	30.70	61.40	40.80	61.50	42.10	17.10	88
Urban slums	44.70	82.70	41.30	82.70	37.90	51.70	29
Urban	24.30	69.20	25.20	68.40	28.40	34.10	123
House	**						
Kachcha	31.40	75.00	27.00	75.00	31.30	27.10	48
Semi-pucca	33.80	67.60	47.80	67.60	47.90	28.20	71
Pucca	25.60	65.30	26.40	64.40	28.10	32.20	121
Current Age	**	**		**		**	
19-24	18.60	70.30	22.30	70.40	22.20	5.60	54
25-29	32.60	73.50	37.30	74.70	39.70	15.70	83
30-34	19.70	68.70	29.50	64.70	31.40	43.10	51
35-39	27.80	55.50	38.90	44.40	38.90	11.10	18
40+	20.00	80.00	20.00	80.00	26.70	33.30	34
Husband's Age	*	*		**	*		
19-24	0.00	66.70	0.00	66.60	0.00	0.00	6
25-29	24.60	70.20	26.40	70.10	24.60	8.80	57
30-34	33.40	70.60	41.40	71.90	45.40	14.70	75
35-39	17.60	70.20	24.60	66.70	26.30	36.80	57
40+	28.60	64.30	42.90	64.30	42.80	35.70	14
Duration of Marriage				*			
<3	0.00	50.00	0.00	50.00	0.00	0.00	4
3-8	25.80	68.00	27.80	67.00	27.90	17.50	97
8-13	25.00	69.10	33.80	69.10	38.20	17.60	68
13-18	29.10	77.50	38.70	77.40	38.70	35.50	31
18+	32.50	60.00	42.50	60.00	45.00	17.50	40

Contd...

Contd...

Caste	**	**		**			
General	35.10	43.40	38.30	43.20	40.00	20.00	60
SC	19.90	88.30	20.00	88.30	21.70	30.00	60
ST	21.70	70.00	43.20	70.00	46.70	15.00	60
OBC	30.00	70.00	30.00	68.40	30.00	13.30	60
Family							
Nuclear	32.90	67.90	40.60	67.20	42.00	21.70	143
Joint	17.50	68.00	21.60	68.00	23.00	14.40	97
Husband's Occupation	*	**		*			
Own business	25.40	65.70	25.40	63.30	26.60	22.80	79
Service	29.70	62.90	32.50	64.00	35.20	11.10	108
Agriculture	22.70	81.20	45.30	81.20	45.30	32.10	53
Wife's Occupation	**						
Own business	52.00	48.00	52.00	48.00	52.00	16.00	25
Service	25.40	76.20	25.40	72.80	27.30	43.60	55
Agriculture	9.70	87.20	22.60	87.10	25.80	58.10	31
Housewife	26.40	63.70	35.00	64.40	36.40	0.00	129
Monthly Income		*		**		**	
<2000	19.40	80.60	27.80	80.60	27.80	13.90	36
2000-5000	27.40	71.80	37.10	72.70	39.50	14.50	124
5000-8000	35.80	54.70	35.70	54.70	38.10	21.40	42
8000-11000	10.00	90.00	10.00	90.00	10.00	40.00	10
11000+	25.00	46.40	25.00	39.40	25.00	39.30	28
Type of Marriage							
Love marriage	27.30	57.70	27.30	57.60	33.40	12.10	33
Arranged marriage	26.50	69.60	33.80	69.10	34.80	20.80	207
Total							240

* Chi-square is significant at the 0.05 level.
** Chi-square is significant at the 0.01 level.

avoidance not only from their in-laws but also from their relatives. Females who were in service faced more negative behaviour by their in-laws than their husbands. The couples, earning more than Rs 11,000 per month faced less quarrels and avoidance from their parents and relatives.

SUMMARY

In most families, when childlessness is a problem, the wife is the first to present herself to the physician. It was also found that some of the couples never went to medical examination although they were worried about the problem.

In case of unexplained childlessness, respondents consult medical experts ranging from simple physicians to infertility experts.

Couples engaged in agriculture found it difficult to reveal about medical confirmation to their husbands and in-laws, as they were afraid of serious consequences.

Along with medical treatment, respondents try non-medical treatment that includes consulting astrologers, saints, magico-spiritual healers, visiting various shrines, following religious practices, etc. These people believe in some external forces operating on them.

It is clear that men are hesitant to get their barrenness tested. Thus, it is clear that a male chooses his place of first medical check-up on the basis of monthly income condition also. It was found that the working women choose private clinics as their first place of check-up.

It was found that respondents changed their eating habits according to the medical treatment or on what was advised. Due to the family pressure, religious sentiments, self-beliefs, women are more prone to change their eating habits.

In the present age, on one hand, moral and social standards are being avoided and things like surrogate motherhood are being given recognition and on the other, there are people who hesitate to use scientific means and prefer to fast and perform many other rituals to obtain a child. They believe that a child should only be born naturally.

When questioned about the replacement of man or woman for a fixed tenure, nearly all the couples said that this kind of practice is only possible in the western countries and will be considered as a sin in the Indian society. The present study reveals that the childless couples need a child so badly that they agreed to do anything whether ethical or not to get a child.

Gender difference was seen in the fact that parents and relative found it easier to put the blame on females and they were more negative towards the female. Co-workers of females remained more indifferent as compared to males. Sometimes they avoided situations which could make childless females uncomfortable.

References

Action Research and Training for Health (ARTH) (2001). Social Influences and Health Seeking Behaviour. *Reproductive Health on the Ground.* A published project report.

Harrison, M. (1964). *A Couples Guide to Cause and Treatments.* Houghton Mifflin Company, Boston.

Mathur, Neeta (1989). *A Psychological Study of Infertile Women.* Ph.D. thesis in Psychology. Mohan Lal Sukhadia University, Udaipur.

Ramu, G.N. (1988). Family Structure Infertility. *Values Concerning Children and Fertility Behaviour*. Sage Publications, New Delhi.

Tyler, Edward T. (1961). *Sterility: Office Management of Infertile Couples.* McGraw Hill Book Company Inc., New York.

Williams, W.W. (1964). *Sterility: The Diagnostic Survey of the Infertile Couples.* Published by W.W. Williams, Magnolia Terrace, USA.

6

Tension Management Processes

When a couple does not have a child within a specific period, it leads to anxiety and loss of self-esteem. A number of psychological and social problems arise due to the lacuna as the couple feels some sort of deficiency within themselves. Though the wife is blamed more than the husband for this deficiency, both the partners may be equally responsible for it. Either of the partners may have the feeling of inadequacy, inferiority, etc. Initially, there may be a feeling of anxiety in all the family members along with the couple. When it is investigated and known with whom the defect lies, the anxiety gets accumulated and intensified within him or her as the case may be, and this adds to the different aspects of the problem. People who have been self-defected, been in control of their lives and believe that hard work leads to success in all tasks, are devastated by infertility experience. Despite the enormous price they pay in terms of money, time, persistence commitment to a schedule, and sacrifice to self and marriage, they cannot do what everyone else can do with a little effort – get pregnant. Competence in this task is beyond their grasp, no matter what they do or how hard they try. This failure invades all aspects of their lives. Couples undergoing any type of treatment, when realise that it is taking too much time and that they are not conceiving according to their plan, begin to worry more and start 'trying harder' to contact the physicians. The impact of infertility is usually far greater on them, and they wonder, what is wrong with them that they cannot do something as natural and as simple as getting pregnant. The lives of the patients begin to revolve around conceiving by following a physician's game plan. The couples focus their attention on what they have failed to accomplish, and soon start neglecting the other goals and needs of their lives.

Childless couples often focus their attention on their failure and when this is done, they undergo different types of losses, i.e., loss of relationship, loss of health, loss of status or prestige, loss of self-esteem, loss of self-confidence, loss of security, loss of fantasy and loss of something or someone of great symbolic value. One of the respondents stated:

> I lost self-confidence; I felt I was no longer attractive. I was in a black mood, particularly when my periods were slightly delayed, which I always interpreted as pregnancy.

These different types of losses help to precipitate depression in the individuals. They are very complex and simultaneous. The losses may be compared to death and divorce. The bereaved relatives and friends of a dead person get a support from the rituals and the funeral. For the infertile couples, there are no rituals. They are not considered bereaved, so they suffer alone. This phenomenon, that there are so many simultaneous losses, and no ritualised support or outlet for the grief, leads to intense tension.

Opinions may vary about what causes tensions. It may be considered as a major life experience, which creates the need for change in a person's life. Tension may also be seen as a prolonged series of day-to-day hassles. Infertility is made stressful due to both the reasons. As a major life event, it involves various types of losses, which contribute to depression. The couples lose balance in their lives. There is, instead, hope one week, grief the next. This cycle creates a very confusing roller coaster with depression, anger and guilt as part of its down side.

Loss of significant relationship is an unspoken fear. Because both the man and woman are hurting, tired and under great pressure they feel depleted of physical and emotional energy. They may become less able to fulfil each other's needs and thereby suffer a loss of closeness to the point of feeling worlds apart.

People take parenthood as much for granted as birth and death. They are born, get an education, then a job, followed by marriage, parenthood and finally death. This is some kind of unwritten cosmic schedule that humans follow and no one really thinks about the progression of events as they live their lives, just flow from one phase of life to another in a seamless fashion. For couples who discover that they cannot have children for whatever reason, the loss of parenthood, a basic ingredient of life, comes as a rude shock. These couples often slip into a deep depression. They sometimes realise that there is no point beating them up pointlessly, about something that is beyond their control. However, couples pass through many agonising hours of self-doubt and despair before they reach the ideal state of acceptance.

Pathways of gender identity are always influenced by cultural context, in western countries and developing ones alike. Despite constraints, however, women do not simply follow cultural plots in restoring their lives. Encountering infertility, they interpret it and compose lives that adapt to, resist, and sometimes reach beyond the master narrative of motherhood. Infertility is positioned differently in older women's lives, compared to younger ones (Mishler, 1999). In many societies, this can be seen that childlessness disqualifies infertile women from part of the "in-group of mothers".

Infertile women were frequently treated by women with children as second class citizens. Thus, infertile women felt more isolated than their partners did as if their lack of children makes it more difficult for them to maintain the same sex friendship. The differential meaning traditionally associated with motherhood versus fatherhood may explain why infertility has a large impact on women's global well-being as compared to men's (Miall, 1985). There is a stigma associated with involuntary childlessness. Physically infertile women felt more stigmatised, physically fertile women with infertile husbands were found with a courtesy stigma, they more actively managed information to protect their husbands from the stigma associated with sexual dysfunction. Various strategies that respondents used to manage potentially stigmatising information included selective concealment, therapeutic and preventive disclosure, medical disclaimers, deviance avowal and a process of practised deception (Miall, 1994).

The cultural ramification and experiences of infertile women in Cameroon, India, Egypt and the US were studied. It demonstrated that anxiety and fear, normative pressure to conceive social stigmatisation and exhaustive searchers for therapy usually marked infertility for women, which tend to be ritualistic, risky, and ethically complex. Infertility often affected women's moral identities and the local moral worlds in which they live (Inhorn, 1994).

Majority of respondents feel that the experience of motherhood was an inherent need and necessity and it gave them higher status in the society. Maximum number of respondents reported childlessness as a biological condition that could be corrected through medical treatment (Deoder, 1995). Most of the couples experience the feelings of loneliness, frustration, rejection and many are also suffering from loss of concentration, sleeplessness, tensions and few also from psychosomatic illness. Childlessness may be said to be a traumatic experience for the couple. A majority of individuals had an accurate understanding of their spouses' feelings related to childlessness (Sheshadri, 1990).

Childlessness leads to a number of simultaneous and complex losses. The experience of infertility involved loss of status and prestige, loss of self-esteem, loss of fantasy, loss of something or someone of great symbolic value (Mahalstedt, 1992).

COPING MECHANISM STUDIES

Coping mechanisms were more frequently adopted by those respondents who had positive attitude towards life. A few couples understood the broader meaning of life and compromised with the situation. They made themselves busy in other activities. They were of the opinion that they would not want to waste their whole life in frustration and depression, but they wanted to make best use of their lives. Some of them kept them busy with the children of neighbours, relatives, friends or of extended family members. Some others had joined social service.

Many of the respondents turned towards religion to cope up with the situation of childlessness. They started believing in religion and started performing religious activities like praying, going on pilgrimage, and performing rituals, reading religious books. Those couples who had positive attitude towards the problem of infertility were found to be well adjusted in their families, workplaces and society and those who had negative attitude towards the problem were found to be maladjusted.

Too many people think infertility is all in their head. Unfortunately, the diagnosis seems to have great popularity with the general public. Some fertile people who are doing their best to avoid pregnancy find it hard to believe that anyone has difficulty becoming pregnant. So, they offer their ill-founded advice, "It must be all in your head" (Harrison, 1964).

There are some couples who, even many years after their unsuccessful treatment, do not try to solve their infertility crisis by any other means. They have no solutions. They still hope or want to do whatever possible to succeed with a pregnancy. The couple's inability to conceive or to achieve a pregnancy, and to experience parenthood, when it is truly desired implies that they suffer a great toll in their quality of life. They are unable to achieve their life expectations or those, which they think society requires from them, thus having a considerable stress imposed on them.

There may be couples who may have practised contraception for some time before trying to conceive and may have regrets at this delay. They may also harbour guilt feelings, especially if an earlier unplanned pregnancy was terminated. These are often telling contributory factors in the development of psychosexual problems among the infertile couples.

There is individual difference among the people, and all the reactions of all the infertile cannot be generalised. There may be some people who are temperamentally grown up or matured enough to be able to make up a satisfactory adjustment in their married life even under difficult infertile situation, whereas there may be those, who, because of their immaturity and lack of understanding, disturb their peaceful and well-settled marital adjustment. Such couples appear to be less task-oriented and less effective in coping with their infertility problem. There is a defence-oriented approach applied by both the partners or by any one of them and they often quarrel and blame each other for their childlessness. There is a tendency to deny the fact of infertility in a vague hope of conceiving in some way or the other in the near future. Infertility may lead to suspiciousness, jealousy, selfishness, stubbornness, irresponsibility and insomnia in the males as well as the females.

Acceptance of being childless is sometimes hampered by the persistent hope of a miracle. When the couples still have hope of conceiving when they cannot, the crisis of infertility becomes worse than before and it evokes many feelings in the couple. Many infertile men and sometimes women also use alcohol for the so-called release of tension of being childless. According to Rouche, it has the power to relieve tension and to satisfy man's need to obtain occasional release from the intolerable clutch of reality. The alcohol addict person drinks for pleasure, whereas a depressed person, as an infertile one, escapes the unavoidable conditions and tries to forget his sorrow by drinking. Such people appear to be immature and dependent individuals with a high level of aspirations. Whereas alcohol induced in most people a feeling of warmth, well-being and general exhilaration, it is not as often thought, a stimulant, but a cerebral depressant. Such relief as its use may bring results from stifling self-criticism and the voice of conscience (Mathur, 1989).

A study was initiated to describe actions that childless couples had taken to help them cope with their feelings and experiences related to childlessness. It was found that respondents used a variety of strategies to cope with infertility. In most cases, the subjects initiated the coping actions to assist themselves in managing their fears, anxiety and disappointments. In some situations, they took measures to increase the space or distance themselves from any reminder of their infertility. At other times, they gave in to their feelings or looked for a hidden meaning of their suffering. Regaining control and being the best were additional coping actions that helped the subjects to improve their self-esteem and decrease their feelings of powerlessness. The subjects also focussed on sharing the burden of infertility by sharing their feelings and experiences with others. The women reported that sharing their feelings and concerns with husbands, friends, relatives and especially other infertile couples proved helpful. Unfortunately, none of the subjects stated that health care providers helped them to cope (Debra et al., 1991).

It was also found that majority of the respondents noticed a change in their behaviour and personality. They became angrier and more frustrated. Most of the women felt that keeping themselves occupied through jobs, hobby activities and work helped them to cope with infertility. Majority of the respondents was aware of different forms of treatment for childlessness and they expressed a high hope in the success of medical treatment. For most of the respondents, child adoption was a lesser-preferred alternative in comparison to the treatment. Some of the respondents were aware of the opinion that they would never opt for child adoption. If they decided to adopt in future the preference would be given to the girl child of the same religion and for unrelated adoption (Deodar, 1995).

ADOPTION

Adoption of children is not a new phenomenon in India. It dates back to ancient days when children, especially the male ones were adopted into the families and given the recognition of natural children. There are many instances found from the ancient Indian texts where people have been denied a child, particularly a male one, resorted to adopting a son of the nearest kith and kin. It is also true that within her new family the young wife does not easily find a secure place or comfortable status until she bears a child, preferably a son. A woman's fear of barrenness is all pervasive. No marital union is thought to be really complete unless it is blessed with a son. If it seems clear that a couple will not produce a son, then usually a boy is adopted. Frequently he will be the child of a relative, a youngster who is an orphan or whose own parents are indigent or have several sons of their own. More rarely, a man may take a second wife if his first does not bear a male child. Divorce is not sanctioned by the sacred writings; among orthodox Indians, marriage is for eternity whether the union proves fecund or barren (Ruth, 1959).

An adopted child is given the rights and privileges of a natural born child. He is given the protection of a home, economic security and can eventually become the heir to the family property. Thus, adoption is to be regarded as the most complete means whereby family life can be restored to a child deprived of its natural family, and the parental instincts of a couple, who cannot have their own child, can be fulfilled.

There is a general widespread impression that infertile couples who adopt often subsequently have children of their own. Several authors have studied this notion and conflicting results have been found. Over-concentration on trying to become pregnant and delay in achieving pregnancy can produce a state of hopelessness and depression that diminishes the chance of conception. In some such cases, tension is relaxed as soon as the woman's name is entered on the list for a curettage, or in others directly a decision is made to adopt, she conceives (Harrison, 1964).

In some other studies only a small percentage of the couples was found to have their own child after adopting one, where a cause and effect relationship might have been obtained between adoption and pregnancy. According to another study, no evidence was found to support the hypothesis that adopting a child in and for itself enhances the possibility that the adoptive couple will conceive. Regarding the treatment of infertility, it is one of the main responsibilities of the therapist to keep the couple as well informed as possible regarding the progress (or lack of it) in their situation. Even in the most highly motivated cases there must come a time where further treatment would be considered futile. With due regards to age and duration of the problem, the therapist introduces the question of adoption. Often on direct interrogation the couple will state that they had considered adoption but had deferred any inquiries until their infertility investigations had been completed and they were certain that conception was impossible. Far too often they have not given any serious thought to adoption (Mathur, 1989).

The reasons for adoption were studied and it was found that the main reason for adoption was that the couples did not have any child, they wished to have a family, be looked after in old age and wanted security. Besides the above reason some couples wanted to adopt additionally for inheritance and passing on of the family name and property. Other reasons were that some couples wanted a boy or a girl depending on which sex they did not have to complete the family. Some couples wanted to replace a dead child, besides the reasons given earlier. The most important reason was that of couples who wanted a child for itself, to have family satisfaction of parental needs. Thus, the child was wanted for itself and not for any benefits that may come to the parents from it (Billimoria, 1984).

PERIOD OF TENSION

On asking the respondents about the longevity of the period of tension caused by childlessness, the Table 6.1 shows that most of the respondents (80%), remained in tension even after four years. But there are very few respondents (3%), who within two years compromised with the situation. Such cases included the respondents who are childless due to the sterility of any one partner. They do not want to embrace any other remedy and some of them cannot afford modern means due to financial problems. About 17 per cent couples have been in tension for two to four years. Most of the couples are those who have had a married life of less than four years and are all under tension. But some respondents decide to adopt a child and therefore come out of these tensions. Surprisingly, the couples under tension within first two years of marriage are from urban settings and reside in *pucca* houses. The knowledge of complications during pregnancy makes them aware of this problem. But tension for more than four years is mostly found in rural couples (83%) and those living in *kachcha* houses (90%).

The data on duration of marriage reveals, the couples (87%) having a married life of 13 to 18 years; 87 per cent couples remain in tension for more than 4 years. Their growing age or crossing the fertility age and less possibility of having a child add greatly to their tension. In the same way, caste also affects the period of tension. Tension was not reported for the first two years of marriage among scheduled castes and scheduled tribes. Their working conditions are such that if within the first two years of marriage, they do not have a child, no tension is

Table 6.1
Period of Tension Caused by Childlessness
Percentage Distribution of Couples by Selected Background Characteristics

Characteristics	*First 2 Years*	*2-4 Years*	*4 + Years*	*Total Per cent*	*Number*
Residence					
Rural	0.00	17.00	83.00	100.00	88
Urban slums	0.00	20.70	79.30	100.00	29
Urban	4.90	16.30	78.80	100.00	123
House					
Kachcha	0.00	10.40	89.60	100.00	48
Semi-pucca	0.00	22.50	77.50	100.00	71
Pucca	5.00	16.50	78.50	100.00	121
Duration of Marriage					
<3	0.00	100.00	0.00	100.00	4
3-8	5.20	14.40	80.40	100.00	97
8-13	1.50	16.20	82.30	100.00	68
13-18	0.00	12.90	87.10	100.00	31
18+	0.00	20.00	80.00	100.00	40
Caste					
General	3.30	5.00	91.70	100.00	60
SC	0.00	8.30	91.70	100.00	60
ST	0.00	30.00	70.00	100.00	60
OBC	6.70	25.00	68.30	100.00	60
Family					
Nuclear	3.50	18.90	77.60	100.00	143
Joint	1.20	12.80	86.00	100.00	97
Husband's Occupation					
Own business	2.50	20.30	77.20	100.00	79
Service	3.70	10.20	86.10	100.00	108
Agriculture	0.00	16.70	83.30	100.00	53
Wife's Occupation					
Own business	8.00	0.00	92.00	100.00	25
Service	5.50	18.20	76.30	100.00	55
Agriculture	0.00	29.00	71.00	100.00	31
Housewife	0.80	17.20	82.00	100.00	129
Total	2.50	17.10	80.40	100.00	240

caused. But the first two years are considered important for producing a child in the general and other backward class category and so if a child is not produced in the first two years, tensions arise. In the general category, 92 per cent couples have been found to be undergoing tensions for more than four years.

If the occupational status of the couple is studied, it is observed that the men and women, who have their own business or are in service, remain tense in the first two years. Men and women in labour or agriculture and housewives mostly live in tension for more than four years. This reveals that the occupation affects the awareness and the seriousness toward this situation.

FEMALE TENSION RELEASE

An attempt was made to ask the female respondents as to what efforts are made by them to get rid of tension. The association of efforts made by them was tested on various background variables. Among the female respondents (n=240), the highest percentage (86) is of those women who totally engross themselves in the household chores so that they have no time to think about their problem (Table 6.2).

Nearly 42 per cent women get involved in social work. One-fourth women consider joining a service and around the same number of women start their own business. Childlessness is a problem, which neither can be shunned off the mind, nor does it go unnoticed. Yet, one out of every three women pursues further studies.

A variety of decisions were observed on the basis of the nature of residence. About 40 per cent women living in cities keep the tension off their heads through service. And 90 per cent women of urban slums get engrossed in the household chores. Also, the highest percentage of women engaged in social work resides in the slums. More than half of the women living in *pucca* houses pursue further studies and 43 per cent women get involved in social work.

Table 6.2

Efforts Made to Get Rid of Tension (Female)
Percentage Distribution of Couples by Selected Background Characteristics (Multiple Choice—'Yes' Responses)

Characteristics	Service	Further Studies	Busy in Household Work	Own Business	Social Work	Number
Residence	**	**				
Rural	8.00	27.30	81.80	17.00	40.90	88
Urban slums	17.20	17.20	89.70	34.50	48.30	29
Urban	40.70	47.20	88.60	26.80	40.70	123
House	**	**				
Kachcha	14.60	14.60	81.30	29.20	41.70	48
Semi-pucca	12.70	25.40	88.70	25.40	39.40	71
Pucca	38.00	51.20	86.80	21.50	43.00	121
Current Age	**		**	**	*	
19-24	14.80	44.40	85.20	11.10	29.60	54
25-29	18.10	31.30	85.50	27.70	39.80	83
30-34	47.10	43.10	88.20	19.60	43.10	51
35-39	44.40	27.80	61.10	16.70	44.40	18
40+	20.60	29.40	100.00	47.10	61.80	34
Duration of Marriage				**		
<3	0.00	50.00	100.00	0.00	50.00	4
3-8	27.80	42.30	82.50	21.60	38.10	97
8-13	27.90	39.70	89.70	19.10	30.90	68
13-18	22.60	16.10	80.60	19.40	51.60	31
18+	22.50	30.00	92.50	45.00	60.00	40
Caste	**	**				
General	31.70	53.30	90.00	20.00	40.00	60
SC	38.30	35.00	90.00	15.00	50.00	60
ST	13.30	26.70	76.70	35.00	38.30	60
OBC	20.00	30.00	88.30	26.70	38.30	60
Husband's Occupation	**	**	**	**		
Own business	34.20	40.50	93.70	30.40	38.00	79
Service	30.60	45.40	84.30	19.40	46.30	108
Agriculture	3.80	11.30	79.20	24.50	37.70	53

Contd...

Contd...

Wife's Occupation	**	**		**		
Own business	0.00	20.00	88.00	92.00	44.00	25
Service	96.40	72.70	87.30	7.30	40.00	55
Agriculture	0.00	0.00	80.60	32.30	41.90	31
Housewife	0.00	32.60	86.80	16.30	41.90	129
Monthly Income	**	**		**	*	
<2000	8.30	8.30	83.30	16.70	38.90	36
2000-5000	16.90	25.00	87.90	21.80	34.70	124
5000-8000	38.10	61.90	81.00	45.20	54.80	42
8000+	57.90	71.10	89.50	15.80	70.00	38
Total	25.80	36.30	86.30	24.20	41.70	240

* Chi-square is significant at the 0.05 level.
** Chi-square is significant at the 0.01 level.

The age of a woman adequately affects her efforts to get rid off the tension. Women (45%) between the age group of 19-24 years pay more attention to further studies, whereas, those who are in the age group of 35-39 years either go for service or for social work. Only 17 per cent women start their own business. All women above the age of forty years engross themselves fully in the household chores. They do it because they do not want to loose their importance and significance in the family.

Women who have had married life less than three years, consider the household chores as an ideal means to avoid their tension. As many as 50 per cent women continue their studies and the rest take up social work. Those who are married for 8 to 13 years have comparatively shown less interest in social work. And 60 per cent women are such who have had a child even after 18 years of marriage, get engaged in social work.

Caste has had a special effect on the service and further studies of childless women. More than half of the women of the general category want to continue their studies and build up their career, and thus want to stay away from the tension of childlessness. One-third women are working (service) and remain busy, whereas, 35 per cent women of the scheduled tribes category are engaged in business of their own.

A great effect of the occupational status of the husband and wife is evident. Women whose husbands are having their own business have been found to have a greater influence towards service and further studies as compared to those whose husbands are engaged in agricultural work. Similarly, women whose husbands are in service, more than half of them opted for further studies and one-third joined some service. The highest percentage (46%), was of those who were engaged in social work and their husbands are in service.

Out of the women, engaged in service, 96 per cent had started working to get rid off the tensions. As much as 87 per cent is getting engrossed in the household chores whereas 92 per cent of women from among those who have their own business run their business to avoid tension. Effect of the family income has also been noticed on the means of warding off tension by women. Families with an income of Rs 2,000 lay more stress on their own business than further studies and also social work is comparatively lesser in vogue. Nearly 70 per cent women of the families with an income of Rs 8,000 or more consider social work to be more effective and more than 70 per cent women lay more stress to further studies and 58 per cent women are working. Thus, it is clear that the family income affects the thinking of the couples. All the answers were put to chi-square test and the significant difference at .01 level is indicated by ** and significant difference at .05 level is indicated by *.

CHANGE IN DAILY ROUTINE

The expression of the mentality and reactions of a man and a woman are very different. Their attitudes towards childlessness are also found to be different. After waiting for a long time to have a child, daily routine of childless couples undergo changes. These changes have been shown through certain scales. Men and women were separately questioned about participation in religious activities and it was found that participation in religious activities has seen a rise among males. Whereas 85 per cent men say that they take more participation, 78 per cent women report in a similar manner. Men take more interest in social activities as compared to women but only half of the men believe that there has been a rise in the participation in social activities due to childlessness and the rest of them report of no such rise (Table 6.3).

Table 6.3
Comparative Changes in Daily Routine
Percentage Distribution of Couples by Selected Background Characteristics

Changes	*Male*			*Female*		
	Increase	*No Change*	*Decrease*	*Increase*	*No Change*	*Decrease*
Participation in religious activities	85.00	13.80	1.30	77.50	18.30	4.20
Participation in social activities	56.30	42.10	1.70	41.30	55.40	3.30
Time spent with spouse	26.70	33.30	40.00	26.70	33.30	40.00
Time spent with family	9.60	36.30	54.20	8.80	37.10	54.20
Interaction with relatives	10.80	35.80	53.30	10.00	37.10	52.90
Time spent on entertainment	30.80	27.90	41.30	24.60	30.00	45.00
Time spent outside home	70.00	21.30	8.80	41.30	39.60	19.20

Childlessness has an adverse effect on the marital life of the couples. This is proved as 40 per cent couples do agree that there is a reduction in the time spent with their spouse, only one-third couples report of no change. Not only has the time spent with the spouses undergone reduction but also the time spent with the rest of the family members has greatly reduced. Less than 10 per cent couples spend more time with the family members and more than 54 per cent couples report of a reduction in the time spent with family members. The time-to-time discussion about children, or the tensions as a result of talks with close relatives may be some of the factors, which lead to such a harsh and rude behaviour of the couple.

Interactions with relatives have also reduced. One-third couples had no change in their relations with their relatives, whereas more than half of the couples want to spend their time in religious and social activities, not with relatives. Difference has been observed in the behaviour of men and women with respect to time spent on entertainment. Nearly 31 per cent men have increased their time of entertainment and 70 per cent men have increased the time spent outside home. On the contrary, 40 per cent women bring no change in the time spent outside home and one out of every five such women spend more time than before in their house. This is the reason, why 45 per cent women have reduced their time spent on entertainment.

It is therefore clear that men are more successful in warding off tensions due to childlessness because women can neither move out of their house nor do their husbands spend time with them as before.

HUSBAND-WIFE SOCIAL ACTIVITIES

Childless couples were asked about their association with social welfare activities and 56 per cent men and 42 per cent women related about their associations. On being asked in detail it was found that they perform acts of social well-being in many ways. Due to childlessness, affectionate behaviour towards orphans has been found mostly in men. More than 20 per cent men help orphans whereas only 13 per cent women do the same. Women have a deep longing for a child of their own to the extent that they do not understand the need of helping orphaned children. An attitude of helping destitute children has also mostly been found in men. About 18 per cent men and 11 per cent women help destitute children. Women, comparatively, take more interest in contributing clothes, medicines and food, etc., to charitable organisation and about 30.8 per cent women do so. But the participation of men is even greater in this field, i.e., about 41.3 per cent (Table 6.4).

Table 6.4
Comparative Association with Social Activities
Percentage Distribution of Couples by Selected Background Characteristics

Association with Social Activity	*Male*		*Female*	
	Yes	*No*	*Yes*	*No*
Helping the destitute	21.30	78.80	13.30	86.70
Helping the poor children	17.90	82.10	11.30	88.80
Helping any organisation	41.30	58.80	30.80	69.20
Donation	33.30	66.70	23.30	76.70
Total	56.30	43.70	41.70	58.30

One-third men are also first in giving offerings and donations whereas less than a fourth women do this. These facts reveal that the attitude of donating money is comparatively lesser in women than in men. Men spend money for social causes with a free-hand whereas women do hold religious feelings, sympathy and pity in their hearts but hesitate to spend money for this; the paternal system of family may be one of the reason for this, because since the beginning women never had the right to spend money and therefore this feeling has indirectly taken hold of them.

FUTURE PLANNING

During the study, an attempt was made to ask all the sterile and infertile couples about their future planning. The answers given by them have been tested on the basis of various variables and using Chi-Square, the significant difference has also been found out. If the decisions taken by the couples are significant and at .01 level, the are shown by ** and significant difference at .05 level has been shown by * (Table 6.5).

Out of all the 240 respondents, more than 55 per cent are those who still wanted to be treated medically. Most of them have been married for less than eight years. About 20 per cent couples now want to compromise with the situation. They

Table 6.5

Future Planning

Percentage Distribution of Couples by Selected Background Characteristics

Characteristics	*No More Treatment*	*More Treatment*	*Adopt*	*Test-tube baby*	*Total Per cent*	*Number*
Residence						
Rural	20.50	59.10	12.40	8.00	100.00	88
Urban slums	31.00	45.00	13.70	10.30	100.00	29
Urban	17.10	56.00	16.30	10.60	100.00	123
House	**	*				
Kachcha	8.30	66.70	14.60	10.40	100.00	48
Semi-pucca	35.20	45.00	9.90	9.90	100.00	71
Pucca	15.70	57.80	17.40	9.10	100.00	121
Current Age	**	**	**			
19-24	0.00	92.60	3.70	3.70	100.00	54
25-29	9.60	52.00	22.70	15.70	100.00	83
30-34	23.50	45.10	21.60	9.80	100.00	51
35-39	33.30	55.60	0.00	11.10	100.00	18
40+	64.70	23.60	8.80	2.90	100.00	34
Husband's Age	**	**		*		
19-24	16.70	83.30	0.00	0.00	100.00	6
25-29	0.00	78.90	12.30	8.80	100.00	57
30-34	14.70	52.00	14.60	18.70	100.00	75
35-39	14.00	57.90	24.60	3.50	100.00	57
40+	64.40	24.40	6.80	4.40	100.00	14
Duration of Marriage	**	**	**			
<3	0.00	100.00	0.00	0.00	100.00	4
3-8	2.10	80.40	7.20	10.30	100.00	97
8-13	16.20	36.80	33.80	13.20	100.00	68
13-18	32.30	51.50	6.50	9.70	100.00	31
18+	62.50	27.50	7.50	2.50	100.00	40
Caste	*					
General	26.70	53.30	11.70	8.30	100.00	60
SC	10.00	55.00	21.70	13.30	100.00	60
ST	28.30	55.00	11.70	5.00	100.00	60
OBC	15.00	60.00	13.30	11.70	100.00	60

Contd...

Contd...

Family	**	**		*		
Nuclear	25.90	51.00	16.80	6.30	100.00	143
Joint	11.30	62.90	11.40	14.40	100.00	97
Husband's Occupation	*	*				
Own business	15.20	64.60	10.10	10.10	100.00	79
Service	18.50	56.50	13.90	11.10	100.00	108
Agriculture	30.20	41.50	22.60	5.70	100.00	53
Wife's Occupation	*	**	**			
Own business	32.00	50.00	0.00	18.00	100.00	25
Service	9.10	60.00	20.00	10.90	100.00	55
Agriculture	36.00	35.00	29.00	0.00	100.00	31
Housewife	18.60	58.90	13.20	9.30	100.00	129
Total	20.00	55.80	14.60	9.60	100.00	240

* Chi-square is significant at the 0.05 level.
** Chi-square is significant at the 0.01 level.

want to compromise to escape the possibility of disappointment of childlessness for a long time and also the expensive treatments. In their opinion, there are hundreds of people who have some or the other disability. But they do not end their lives there, they live with it. In the same manner, childlessness should also be considered as a disability. This will help in living a better life.

About 15 per cent couples have decided to stop further treatment and adopt a child. These couples were informally indirectly asked about surrogacy. But some of them do not know about it completely and some totally denied it. A mere percentage of nearly 10 per cent couples were prepared for having a test-tube baby. According to them, giving money and getting their own child, would be the best option they could ever have.

Nearly 35 per cent couples out of all those couples who neither want to go on with further treatment nor feel the need of adopting a child but want to compromise with the situation, live in semi-*pucca* houses. Also, women who are above the age of 40 years, do not want to continue their treatment so the fertility reduces after this age.

Couples with a married life of more than 18 years and mostly scheduled tribe couples have opted for a compromise with the situation and stop further treatment. The nature of family has an evident effect on such decisions because if they have family support, the childless couples remains motivated. This is the reason why treatment is always stressed upon in a joint family even if it is the option of a test-tube baby, but in case of adoption the importance is lesser than that in a nuclear family.

The economic condition of the family definitely affects the decisions of the couple, because 80 per cent couples with an income of more than Rs 8,000 want to continue their treatment and 40 per cent are ready for test-tube baby. After bearing the expenses of medicines and tests, the doctor's fee and other expenses for just the possibility of having a child cannot be afforded by most couples. Another logic has come forth for this that women who have a service, 60 per cent of them want to continue their treatment because they can bear the expenses of their treatment completely or to some extent. Likewise, husband and wife having their own business are prepared to spend more for having a child. Almost 20 per cent business-women are prepared to have a test-tube baby.

Couples who want to adopt a child were asked individually as to what child they would like to adopt – from an orphanage, a poor child or a relative's child, a difference was seen between the opinion of husband and wife.

Men are more interested to adopt a relative's child whereas women find adopting a poor child more appropriate. According to them, adopting a relative's child is always unsafe because the child will always be in contact with the real parents and therefore will never be able to embrace or adjust with the legal parents. Situation of interference in decisions also arises as the rest of the family members are already related to the relative's child. Men are in favour of adopting a relative's child due to factors like purity of blood, and cultural ethical equality. But women wish to have their 'own child' without involving any relation. On raising the topic of adoption from a orphanage, both man and woman remained dumb. When asked informally, some said that it was necessary to know about the caste and the family background of the child. The effect of the environment and nature by birth both build up a child's personality. Therefore, it is not right to take up this risk. Some respondents have made up their mind for adoption but have not decided whose child or from where, they will adopt. Some said, that if given a chance, they will adopt a girl-child so that they will be able to educate her and get her married and thus will fulfil all the family duties and be satisfied. They will spend on her as per their wishes. But if they adopt a boy-child, they will have to spend their entire lifetime with him, even if they do not want to.

EFFECT OF BACKGROUND CHARACTERISTICS ON TENSION MANAGEMENT

The efforts made by couples to get rid of tensions caused by childlessness are shown in Table 6.6. It was found that keeping themselves busy in the household work is the common effort to release the tensions. It was also seen that there were similarities among all the females belonging to different background characteristics. Males were also found keeping busy in household work to release their tensions. Females from urban settings chose service to divert their tensions.

More couples from rural settings wanted to continue their treatments and very few couples residing in semi-*pucca* houses agreed upon adoption of a child. It was another alternative suggested for tension release. Females of 19 to 24 years wanted to continue their treatment and kept themselves busy in household work.

Couples who were married for less than three years did not adopt a child because they had a hope of conception. But after 18 years of marriage only one-fourth of couples continued

Table 6.6

Tension Management

Percentage Distribution of Couples by Selected Background Characteristics

Characteristics	*House-hold Work (Male)*	*House-hold Work (Female)*	*Service (Female)*	*More Treat-ment*	*Adoption*	*No.*
Residence			**			
Rural	40.90	81.80	8.00	59.10	12.40	88
Urban slums	41.40	89.70	17.20	45.00	13.70	29
Urban	37.40	88.60	40.70	56.00	16.30	123
House			**	*		
Kachcha	52.10	81.30	14.60	66.70	14.60	48
Semi-pucca	39.40	88.70	12.70	45.00	9.90	71
Pucca	33.90	86.80	38.00	57.80	17.40	121
Current Age	*	**	**		**	
19-24	29.60	85.20	14.80	92.60	3.70	54
25-29	45.80	85.50	18.10	52.00	22.70	83
30-34	51.00	88.20	47.10	45.10	21.60	51
35-39	38.90	61.10	44.40	55.60	0.00	18
40+	20.60	100.00	20.60	23.60	8.80	34
Husband's Age	*			**	**	
19-24	33.30	100.00	0.00	83.30	0.00	6
25-29	35.10	80.70	15.80	78.90	12.30	57
30-34	42.70	89.30	24.00	52.00	14.60	75
35-39	47.40	80.70	42.10	57.90	24.60	57
40+	28.90	93.30	24.40	24.40	6.80	14
Duration of Marriage	*			**	**	
<3	0.00	100.00	0.00	100.00	0.00	4
3-8	38.10	82.50	27.80	80.40	7.20	97
8-13	51.50	89.70	27.90	36.80	33.80	68
13-18	38.70	80.60	22.60	51.60	6.50	31
18+	25.00	92.50	22.50	27.50	7.50	40

Contd...

Contd...

Caste	**		**			
General	26.70	90.00	31.70	53.30	11.70	60
SC	60.00	90.00	38.30	55.00	21.70	60
ST	33.30	76.70	13.30	55.00	11.70	60
OBC	36.70	88.30	20.00	60.00	13.30	60
Family			**	**		
Nuclear	43.40	88.10	30.10	51.00	16.80	143
Joint	34.40	83.50	19.60	62.90	11.40	97
Husband's Occupation		**	**	*		
Own business	36.70	93.70	34.20	64.60	10.10	79
Service	38.90	84.30	30.60	56.50	13.90	108
Agriculture	43.40	79.20	3.80	41.50	22.60	53
Wife's Occupation	*			**	**	
Own business	40.00	88.00	0.00	50.00	0.00	25
Service	43.60	87.30	96.40	60.00	20.00	55
Agriculture	72.70	80.60	0.00	35.00	29.00	31
Housewife	31.80	86.80	0.00	58.90	13.20	129
Monthly Income	**		**			
<2000	55.60	83.30	8.30	47.20	25.00	36
2000-5000	42.70	87.90	16.90	55.60	14.50	124
5000-8000	33.30	81.00	38.10	59.50	9.50	42
8000-11000	18.40	89.50	57.90	80.00	0.00	10
11000+	21.40	86.10	53.60	53.60	14.30	28
Type of Marriage			*			
Love marriage	36.40	84.80	19.30	72.70	12.10	33
Arranged marriage	39.60	86.50	11.20	53.10	15.00	207
Total						240

* Chi-square is significant at the 0.05 level.
** Chi-square is significant at the 0.01 level.

their treatment but they did not want to adopt a child. When focused on their efforts caste-wise, it was revealed that females of general, scheduled caste and other backward class categories liked and chose to keep them busy in household works. The females of general and scheduled caste category also chose service as a tension management effort.

The type of family also influences the efforts made to get rid of tensions. In the nuclear families, adoption was more preferred than joint families. Males engaged in farming were not found interested in more treatment and they wanted a child by adoption. But females in service were found more interested in further treatment. Since the treatment of sterility and infertility is quite expensive, the couples earning below Rs 2,000 per month did not want more treatment and they wanted to start a new life with an adopted child. According to them, after adoption the child fills the vacuum of life and it was a widely held belief that many times after adoption childless couples would themselves conceive. Couples, who had love marriage and where the wives were in service, they were interested in continued treatment because they could afford the expenses.

SUMMARY

When a couple does not have a child within a specific period, it leads to anxiety and loss of self-esteem. A number of psychological and social problems arise due to the lacuna as the couple feels some sort of deficiency within themselves. Though the wife is blamed more than the husband for this deficiency, both the partners may be equally responsible for it. Those respondents, who had positive attitude towards life, more frequently adopted coping patterns. A few couples understood the broader meaning of life and compromised with the situation. They made themselves busy in other activities. Males were also found keeping busy in household work to release their tensions. Females from urban settings chose service to divert their tensions. Some of them kept themselves busy with the children of neighbours, relatives, friends or of extended family members. Some others had joined social service.

Many of the respondents turned towards religious activities to cope up with the situation of childlessness. They started believing in religion and started performing religious activities like praying, going on pilgrimage, performing rituals and reading religious books. They were found to be better adjusted in their families, workplaces and society and those who had negative attitude towards the problem were found to be maladjusted.

Couples, who have practised contraception for some time before trying to conceive, regret at this delay. They also harbour guilt feelings especially if an earlier unplanned pregnancy was terminated. These are often contributory factors in the development of psychosexual problems among the infertile couples. Couples who were married for less than three years did not adopt a child because they had a hope of conception. But after 18 years of marriage only one-fourth of couples continued their treatment but they did not want to adopt a child.

Some couples have decided to stop further treatment and adopt a child. In the nuclear families, adoption was more preferred than joint families. Males engaged in farming were not found interested in more treatment and they wanted a child by adoption.

These couples were informally indirectly asked about surrogacy. But some of them do not know about it completely and some totally denied it. A small percentage of couples were prepared for having a test-tube baby. According to them, giving money and getting their own child, would be the best option they could ever have.

Men are more interested to adopt a relative's child, whereas women find adopting a poor child more appropriate. There appears to be a great hesitation in adoption of child from orphanage. They consider it necessary to know about the caste and the family background of the child. Some said that if given a chance they will adopt a girlchild so that they will be able to educate her and get her married and thus will fulfil all the family duties and be satisfied. They will spend on her as per their wishes. But if they adopt a boychild, they will have to spend their entire lifetime with him, even if they do not want to.

References

Billimoria, H.M. (1984). *Child Adoption: A Study of Indian Experience.* Himalayan Publications, Mumbai.

Debra, C. et al., (1991). *Coping Strategies of Infertile Women.* Journal of Gynaecology and Neonatal Nursing.

Deodar, S.C. (1995). *Infertility and Adoption Option.* Project report submitted to Tata Institute of Social Science (TISS), Mumbai.

Harrison M. (1964). *A Couple's Guide to Causes and Treatments.* Houghton Mifflin Company, Boston.

Inhorn, M.C. (1994). *Interpreting Infertility: Medical Anthropological Perspective:* Introduction. Social Science and Medicine.

Mahalstedt, P.P. (1992). *The Psychological Component of Infertility.* Fertility and Sterility.

Mathur, Neeta (1989). *A Psychological Study of Infertile Women.* Ph.D. thesis in Psychology. Mohan Lal Sukhadia University, Udaipur.

Miall, C.E. (1985). *The Stigma of Involuntarily Childlessness, Social Problems.* Hemisphere Publishing Company, USA.

Miall, C.E. (1994). *Community Construct of Involuntary Childlessness: Sympathy, Stigma and Social Support.* Canadian Review of Social and Anthropology. Sociology and Anthropology.

Mishler, E.G. (1999). *Storylines: Crafts Artists' Narratives of Identity.* Harvard University Press, Cambridge.

Prabhu, P.N. (1963). *Hindu Social Organisation.* Popular Prakashan, Mumbai.

Ruth, Nanda A. (1959). *The Family: Its Functional Destiny.* Harper and Brothers Publications, New York.

Sheshadri, A. (1990). *Perception of Childless Couples Regarding Childlessness, Treatment and Adoption.* Project report submitted to Tata Institute of Social Science, Mumbai.

7

Social Consequences of Sterility and Infertility

Every human being has an instinctive desire to become a parent and look after the offspring. Being a parent has many rewards and pleasures. For most people, to live without having a child, in spite of having a loving mate, is unthinkable. Parenthood, as a stage of life, is characterised by the need to look after, to take care, to give both materially and in terms of affection. For a woman, it is also an expression of creativity and has both biological and psychological roots.

It is evident from our holy books, old stories and myths, how people were blessed with children after praying and fasting and performing various types of religious rituals. Fecundity or ability to produce children has a positive social value. Procreation is socially desirable for religious and family reasons. Children ensure the continuation of the family lineage. Generally, couples who do not bear children within few years of their marriage start worrying. The inability of the couple, to conceive or produce a live birth, is known as childlessness.

The lack of uniform definitions has hounded research on childlessness while it is clear that infertility childlessness or sterility all refer to the inability of a couple to conceive or bear a child when desired. The actual definition of infertility is somewhat elastic; the classical period of time is usually taken as two years after a healthy marriage, without any contraception. But, in well over half the patients attending an infertility clinic for the first time, the period of infertility, is shorter than this. The relative speed with which the investigations are carried out can be slightly flexible, depending upon both, the age of the patient and the duration of the condition.

Infertility is failure to produce a child. It is slightly different from the term 'sterility' which is inability to conceive and produce a child, where, after all the necessary investigation it has been confirmed that conception is not possible. In the context of the Indian society, if these two terms are viewed from a sociological viewpoint, their definitions clearly bring out their effect. Infertility is a condition in which the woman can conceive but not deliver. She is not considered as *banjh* or 'dry womb'. Her status and situation is not stigmatised in her family, kinship and society. But sterility is 'barrenness'; it is a stigma for her. A woman who can neither give her family an heir nor can bring continuity in the society, is a curse, her life will always be incomplete due to lack of motherhood. Due to her own, or her husband's sterility, she is not considered worthy to attend family, religious or social occasions because her presence on these occasions is considered inauspicious. People even consider looking at her, especially in the morning, as inauspicious. Such a woman is addressed as 'barren', 'dry womb' or a 'cursed womb'. The other women of the family keep their children away from her. They do not let such a woman come in contact with their children, or with their toys and clothes. In fact, this condition gives the actual picture of the childless couple in the family and the society.

Many conditions are known to cause, or to contribute to, childlessness. Contrary to the popular belief that childlessness is due to some physical problem in the woman, when studied scientifically, the causes of childlessness may be found in both men and women. The causes of childlessness can be physical as well as psychological and sexual.

Sometimes, all other factors are positive and yet conception does not take place. This may be due to circumstantial factors like the couples staying together but not having enough privacy for sexual union, the frequency of intercourse not being adequate and appropriate, psychological distance inspite of living together, etc. Such problems are reflected among cases who often seek the help of the counsellor, when on medical investigation all tests give positive results and yet conception does not occur. It is also seen that certain genetic or social factors seem to be correlated with infertility.

Sterility and infertility have negative social values in the Indian culture. Formerly, these were viewed as a disgrace and a mark of shame. In many societies, wife often has no status until she becomes a mother. The infertile couples' relatives and friends do not give genuine support in majority of the cases. Pregnant women and other people's children often evoked negative feelings among women with infertility or sterility.

The social consequences of infertility impose serious emotional effect on the infertile couple, especially, the women. There is social and cultural deprivation, and divorce is its major outcome. The individual finds it difficult to interact with spouse, family, friends and acquaintances. The infertile couples generally lie deliberately, and reject social exchanges. They do not get genuine support from the relatives and friends and have negative feelings towards pregnant women and other's children.

MARITAL LIFE AND FAMILY SITUATIONS

Family is the basic unit of the organisation of human society. If a person wants to understand the formation, administration and working of a social organisation, it is important that he understands family from a sociological point of view. The structure of a family is based on the relationships of kinship, which are linked together in the patterns of duty and rights, feelings and governance. Emotional thoughts like love, cooperation, childbearing, and service are found among the members of the family. In the context of the Indian society, joint family is the smallest sociological unit of the social organisation. It is true that the nature and the working of joint families have changed. Nature of marriages has also undergone changes—late marriages, love marriages and inter-caste marriages are in vogue. Marriage is no longer a relationship between two families but a relationship between individuals. Youngsters sometimes get married with the cooperation of parents but these days, the affirmation and consent of the entire family does not matter much. The new generation does not give much importance to elderly people, they take personal decision and accomplish any big task. The status and image of a person have started affecting his family membership.

Many factors are responsible for such a situation, be it the effect of westernisation and urbanisation, or the effect of education and the industrial age. But, the family scenario in the society is undergoing a rapid change. Decisions like marriage, childbearing, etc., are now made on the basis of logical reasoning. Consequently, the level of satisfaction of the family has also changed; among other decisions, for the good of one's nuclear family, the time of having a child, the number of children, and the gap between each child, are also present. In case of any problem, an attempt is made to solve it by holding discussion between the husband and wife. This condition shows that the role of the family is changing.

Newly married couples may have put off having children for a few years while they were getting settled in their marriage, or their careers. They heard all about accidental pregnancies, so they compulsively chose a method of contraception. One day the time seems right to begin their family and they stop using any birth control method. But the first month the woman, menstruates. Another month goes by, and she menstruates again. They both begin to wonder what is wrong. People tell them not to worry. The next month, and the month afterward pass, and still no pregnancy. It is found that many couples adopt contraception early in their married life and discover a problem only when they discontinue contraception, to have a child (Freedman and Campbell, 1959). Abortion and miscarriages are other causes of childlessness. For the purpose of minimising the size of the family, some couples practice induced abortions. After some period they find that tension and anxiety are overwhelming. They find that their life is filled with fears about what is wrong. Tension and anxiety are not the only reasons to begin thinking about starting an infertility investigation but there are several other reasons for this. The other associated factor is miscarriage, which is more of an accidental abortion. The grief of a woman who has failed to bear a live born child is no less in modern society than it was for our forefathers (Insler, 1981).

A couple's response to childlessness can be understood as both a crisis and a mourning process. Many aspects of the marital relationships are affected profoundly by efforts to come to terms with infertility, sexual identity, self-esteem, communication patterns and futures life choices. Many couples use denial as the first method of coping with infertility, which often prevents them from moving forward in the mourning process. Anger, directed inward in the form of depression and learned helplessness, or outward through expression of rage and bitterness, can lead to depression or emotional isolation. The expression of anger is mixed with the feelings of intense grief and commonly, somatic distress and guilt.

SOCIAL INTERACTIONS AND BEHAVIOUR

The couples viewed bearing and rearing children as a confirmation of one's masculinity and femininity. Procreation, for a male, was a concrete demonstration of his virility and maturity, to self and community. For women bearing children is a demonstration of their fecundity, femininity and conformity to the virtue of motherhood (Mandelbaum, 1970). Infertility affects the couples in a number of ways. The females undergo a conflict over their femininity and fear of reproduction and pregnancy. A man's self-esteem is directly associated with masculinity, and that of a woman with femininity.

When most couples are told that they are infertile they find it difficult to accept this verdict. After all, people all over the world are having babies every minute. It is the most natural thing in the world. The next thought that occurs to them is considering the rate at which medical technology is advancing, surely the problem can be fixed. But there are still some couples who slip through the cracks. After spending a huge amount of money and following all the doctors' instructions, some couples still fail to conceive a child. When it is found that it is very difficult or impossible to conceive, both the partners are under severe stress, and they undergo a situation of helplessness because this stress is found to be unavoidable and they cannot do anything. This helplessness is a learned response in the face of a situation, which cannot be controlled (Mathur, 1989).

It was found that in those cases where the problem was diagnosed in the males, the respondents tried to hide the fact and held women responsible for childlessness. In other cases where females were diagnosed infertile, it was disclosed instantly. Gender difference was seen in the fact that the respondents found it easier to put the blame on women. When couples were asked, whom they held responsible for their childlessness, the responses of husbands and wives were remarkably different.

Infertility affects the marital relationships on aspects such as sexual identity, self-esteem, communication patterns and future life choices (Shapiro and Constance, 1982). After diagnosis the problem or due to delay in pregnancy, major change in the interpersonal relations of couples was observed. Some respondents reported that their relations did not suffer because of infertility but had become more strong. There was no friction due to childlessness.

Infertile couples' relatives and friends did not give genuine support in majority of the cases. During the early years of marriage, the female respondents reported that their family members and relatives were more loving, cooperative and understanding but as the problem was diagnosed, they observed a change in their relationship. Their family members had become quarrelsome, frustrated over small matters and husband had increased alcohol intake and used to stay out of home for a comparatively increased duration. In some cases, the husband avoided the wife's company.

Most of the respondents stopped attending any social gathering where they were reminded of their infertility. They withdrew from people and activities that reminded them of their inability to conceive. They also tried to withdraw from the thought of children, and tried not to think about infertility consciously.

On getting news about pregnancy of some relatives, friends or neighbours, more females as compared to male respondents showed negative responses. They reported that feelings of annoyance, jealousy, misfortune, failure came into their mind.

It was found that some of the female respondents themselves avoided attending such ceremonies because they felt embarrassed and humiliated on such occasions, because people around them passed some remark or the other and they became the topic for gossip and conversation. Some of respondents stated that they were not invited on birthday parties of children, as they did not have children and they knew it very well that participation of childless females in social gatherings especially rituals related to pregnancy or childbirth, was restricted because these women were considered inauspicious or incomplete. They were called at the time of having food but not invited at the time of performance of rituals.

MEDICAL ASSISTANCE AND TREATMENT

In most families, when childlessness is a problem, the wife is the first to present herself to the physician. There still are too many instances where the wife is subjected to extensive studies without any preliminary attention to the fertility status of the husband. In Indian society, husband do not wish to get themselves examined first for childlessness. Even today, in most cases of infertility, it is the woman who seeks help first. But the condition is not confined to women (Harrison, 1964). It was also found that some of the couples never went for medical examination although they were worried about the problem.

In case of unexplained childlessness, respondents consult medical experts ranging from simple physicians to infertility experts. They also visit outstation clinics for better medical treatment and expertise. There are occasions when patients may travel many miles to renowned medical centres. Yet, the investigation of infertility problems has become so common that many patients can be treated in their own local areas.

Many childless female respondents found it difficult to reveal about medical confirmation to their husbands and in-laws, as they were afraid of serious consequences. Male respondents also had the feeling of depression and shock when they heard about the inability of their wives to produce a baby. They became angry with their wives. In other cases, where males were diagnosed infertile, they could not believe it and got very much disappointed. Many respondents believed that medical treatment worked only "if one had good luck and if God wanted to give child to someone". Respondents also took ayurvedic medicines.

Along with medical treatment respondents try non-medical treatment that includes consulting astrologers, saints, magico-spiritual healers, visiting various shrines, following religious practices, etc. There are paranoid symptoms also that are linked to their infertility. They become a bit sensitive and suspicious. They think that someone is behind their inability to conceive. These people believe in some external forces operating on them (Mathur, 1989). Both men and women commonly mentioned supernatural causes. Some women were accused of being witches and were therefore held responsible for their childlessness by their in-laws' family. Jealousy of relatives and neighbours, curses of ancestors, breach of cultural traditions, were also perceived to be the causes of infertility.

Many couples attributed their childlessness to "God's will" or to their destiny. One of the interesting observations in that study was the many of the women did not blame their husbands despite the husband's physical inabilities, but felt that it was their own destiny and that nothing could be achieved against God's will.

The infertile people find it very difficult to talk to other people about their childlessness because of the lack of self-confidence, and because they have suspicion that their neighbours and relatives mock at them behind their backs and abuse them for their inability to conceive.

It is clear that men are hesitant to get their potency tested. It is also clear that a male chooses his place of first medical check-up on the basis of monthly income and economic condition also. It was found that the working women choose private clinics as their first place of check-up.

An Indian woman should be an ideal wife, an ideal daughter-in-law and an ideal mother. She lives her life on this principle. The women face more tensed atmosphere when the report shows their fault.

It was found that one out of ten men changed his eating habits according to the medical treatment or on what he was advised. Due to the family pressure, religious sentiments, self-beliefs, women are more prone to change their eating habits.

With the help of various government organisations and NGOs, allopathy has spread to many villages, and with the help of health camps, satellite hospitals, primary health centres, etc., people have been educated about all the latest diseases, their symptoms and their cures. Yet their faith in alternative therapy is not shaken.

In the present age, on one hand, moral and social standards are being avoided and things like surrogate motherhood are being given recognition. On the other hand, there are people who hesitate to use scientific means and prefer to fast, and perform many other rituals, to obtain a child. They believe that a child should only be born naturally.

When questioned about the replacement of man or woman for a fixed tenure, nearly all the couples said that this kind of practice is only possible in the western countries and will be considered as a sin in the Indian society. The present study reveals that the childless couples need a child so badly that they agreed to do anything whether ethical or not to get a child.

TENSION MANAGEMENT PROCESSES

When a couple does not have a child within a specific period, it leads to anxiety and loss of self-esteem. A number of psychological and social problems arise due to the lacuna as the couple feels some sort of deficiency within themselves. Though the wife is blamed more than the husband for this deficiency, both the partners may be equally responsible for it. When it is investigated and the deficient partner is identified, the anxiety gets accumulated and intensified within him or her as the case may be, and this adds to the different aspects of the problem.

Different types of losses help to precipitate depression in the suffering individuals. They are very complex and simultaneous. The losses may be compared to death and divorce. The bereaved relatives and friends of a dead person get support from the rituals and the funeral. For the infertile couples, there are no rituals. They are not considered bereaved, so they suffer alone. This phenomenon, of so many simultaneous losses, and no ritualised support or outlet for the grief, leads to intense tension.

Loss of significant relationship is an unspoken fear. Because both the man and woman are hurt, tired and under great pressure they feel depleted of physical and emotional energy. They may become less able to fulfil each other's needs and thereby suffer a loss of closeness to the point of feeling worlds apart.

There may be couples who may have practised contraception for some time before trying to conceive and may have regrets at this delay. They may also harbour guilt feelings especially if an earlier unplanned pregnancy was terminated. These are often telling contributory factors in the development of psychosexual problems among the infertile couples.

There are some couples who, even many years after their unsuccessful treatment, do not try to solve their infertility crisis by any other means. They have no solutions. They still hope or want to do whatever possible, to succeed with a pregnancy. The couple's inability to conceive or to achieve a pregnancy, and to experience parenthood, when it is truly desired implies that they suffer a lot in their quality of life. They are unable to achieve their life expectations or those, which they think society requires from them, thus having a considerable stress imposed on them.

Sheshadri (1990) in her study found that childless couples had to listen to the advices, particularly to the taunts, of relatives and others but neither could retort when advised or taunted, as they felt helpless. To find out the solutions of the problem couples also consulted many doctors and most had undergone all the tests related to diagnosis of their problem. A very small minority perceived the treatment to be useful. In fact the couples had many grievances relating to expenditure made and time spent on treatment. Couples in the study had taken several non-medical steps especially religious measures.

Some couples now want to compromise with the situation. They want to compromise, to escape the possibility of disappointment of childlessness for a long time, and also the expensive treatments. In their opinion, there are hundreds of people who have some or the other disability. But they do not end their lives there, they live with it. In the same manner, childlessness should also be considered as a disability. This will help in living a better life.

Some couples have decided to stop further treatment and adopt a child. These couples were informally, indirectly asked about surrogacy. But some of them do not know about it completely and some totally denied it. Only a few couples were prepared for having a test-tube baby. According to them, giving money and getting their own child, would be the best option they could ever have. Men are more interested to adopt a relative's child whereas women find adopting a poor child more appreciable. According to them, adopting a relative's child is always unsafe because the child will always be in contact with the real parents and therefore will never be able to embrace or adjust with the legal parents. Situation of interference in decisions also arises as the rest of the family members are already related to the relative's child. But men are in favour of adopting a relative's child due to factors like purity of blood, and cultural ethical equality. On the other hand, women wish to have their 'own child' without involving any relation. On raising the topic of adoption from a orphanage, both man and woman remained dumb. When asked informally, some said that it was necessary to know about the caste and the family background of the child. The effect of the environment and nature by birth both builds up a child's personality. Therefore, it is not right to take up this risk. Some respondents have made up their mind for adoption but have not decided whose child or from where, they will adopt. Some said, that if given a chance, they would adopt a girl-child so that they will be able to educate her and get her married. Thus, they will fulfil all the family duties and be satisfied. They will spend on her as per their wishes. But if they adopt a boy-child, they will have to spend their entire lifetime with him, even if they do not want to.

The reasons for adoption were studied in 1984 by Billimoria. Demographic profile of couples was obtained from a family welfare agency, in Mumbai. It was found that the main reason for adoption for few couples was that they did not have any child. They wished to have a family, be looked after in old age and wanted security. Besides the above reasons, some couples wanted to adopt additionally for inheritance and passing on of the family name and property. Other reasons were that couples wanted a boy or girl depending on which sex they did not have to complete the family. The most important group was that of a few couples who wanted a child for itself, to have family satisfaction of parental needs. Thus the child was wanted for it and not for any benefits that may come to the parents from it. Another supporting survey for adoption comes from the study of infertile couples' views on adoption and the sample of the study was selected from Ambala district of Haryana. It was found that in all, 108 (84%) couples expressed the desire for a child. Significantly more couples with primary infertility 55 (92%) expressed such a desire compared to 53 couples (77%) with secondary infertility. Among the wives about 71 per cent favoured adoptions, 24 per cent opposed it, and the remaining 6 per cent were not sure of about it. On the other hand, as many as 84 per cent of the husbands favoured adoption; only 14 per cent opposed it and a marginal 2 per cent were equivocal (Singh et al., 1996).

On the other hand, Stewart and Glazer (1986) studied the expectations and coping strategies of women undergoing *in vitro* fertilisation (IVF) treatment. The women reported that having a close relationship with the members of the IVF team helped them to cope with their problem. The women found comfort in knowing that the team members provided them with detailed information concerning IVF and were available on a 24-hour basis to offer support. The women's husbands, who were actively involved in the treatment, both physically and emotionally, also facilitated coping. The husbands took over managing the households, administered the intramuscularly infertility drugs at home and cried with their wives when they were unsuccessful in conceiving. The women reported that sharing their experience with family members or close friends was helpful because they provided understanding and loving support.

SOCIAL CONSEQUENCES OF CHILDLESSNESS

Sterility and infertility have negative social values in the Indian culture. Formerly, these were viewed as a disgrace and a mark of shame. Social consequences of childlessness impose serious emotional effect on the childless couples, especially, the women. Infertile or sterile individuals may undergo a loss of relationship, health, status, prestige, self-esteem, self-confidence, security, fantasy and loss of something or someone of great symbolic value.

In many societies, wife often has no status until she becomes a mother. Infertility had a far more negative influence on the female subjects, behaviour with disappointment, jealousy and marital dissatisfaction. Psychological acceptance of this condition also developed significantly slower in the female group (Brand, 1981). Jacobson and Lalos (1986) concluded that infertile couples undergo grief, depression, guilt and feelings of inferiority and isolations; women openly admitted more symptoms than their partners because infertility was found in them, and marital relationships and sexual life were also affected.

Rosenfeld (1984) found that a woman feels inadequate when she fails at the most critical times. Social interrogations as 'hows' and 'whys' makes the woman feel tense and it reminds her every now and then that she has failed to conceive. Where husbands experienced impotency, Berger (1980) observed that among these couples the women showed anger towards the husband; there were psychiatric symptoms and dreams about their concern for the husband; a wish to be rid of him, and a guilt over this wish. Masters and Johnson (1970) stated that the greatest problems of infertile couples are social and cultural deprivation, the problems of role expectations, and self-image among the couples with nervous system disorders arise and they cannot work through.

In addition to the psychological frustration derived from the inability to fulfil their reproductive preferences, infertile couples are often exposed to a variety of family and social pressure. The infertile couples generally lie deliberately and reject social exchanges. They do not get genuine support from the relatives and friends and have negative feelings towards pregnant women and other's children. Mathur (1989) concluded that there is social and cultural deprivation, and divorce is its major outcome. The individual finds it difficult to interact with spouses, families, friends and acquaintances. Another supporting study for this comes from Lalos et al. (1985) that the infertile couples' relative and friends did not give genuine support in majority of the cases. Pregnant women and other people's children often evoked negative feelings among them. In societies where a woman's identity is closely linked to her maternal role, infertility can lead to social stigmatisation and may adversely affect gender relations, kinship ties, inheritance, and marriage and divorce patterns. Inhorn (1994) stated that infertility affects both men and women of reproductive age. The inability to have children can have profound negative implications for the individual. Sharma (1990) agreed that the divorce rates among infertile marriages were greater than those of couples with children. Divorce rates were higher in urban areas as compared to the rural ones. In contrast to the above Renne (1977) found that the infertile couples had succeeded in living together inspite of a long lasting infertility problem, indicating that their marital relationship has been stable.

TESTING OF HYPOTHESES

> When a woman's identity is closely linked to her maternal role, childlessness can lead to social stigmatisation and may adversely affect gender relations, kinship ties, inheritance, marriage and divorce patterns.

It was evident from the responses that fertility or ability to produce children has a positive social value. Family and society looks down upon the couples' who are not able to bear children. Insensitive behaviour to their childlessness was extended by their family members, neighbours, relatives and friends. They were under constant social pressure from family and society and some women even had to face the threat of remarriage and divorce. Because of such attitudes the childless couples, especially women, felt isolated from family and society; they expressed the feelings of being excluded from couples having children at family gatherings and other social events. Men also reported the feelings of isolation but women reported greater social isolation especially in those cases where family members were not supporting them.

> The wives face more problems of social adjustments, as compared to their husbands.

In the present study, most of the women respondents withdrew from people and activities that reminded them of their inability to conceive. They stopped attending social gatherings where they were reminded of their infertility. Negative emotional responses were reported by majority of wives respondents as compared to their husbands.

Some of the female respondents themselves avoided attending such ceremonies because they felt embarrassed and humiliated on such occasions as people around them passed some remarks or comments and they became the topic for gossip and conversation. Some of respondents stated that they were not invited on birthday parties of children, as they did not have children and they knew it very well that participation of childless females in social gatherings (especially rituals related to pregnancy or childbirth) was restricted because these women were considered inauspicious or incomplete.

Childless males as such did not report any negative reactions for such ceremonies and rituals. It is because perhaps these ceremonies are more female centred and males did not have many roles to perform in these.

> Family members and relatives have more negative attitude towards females as compared to males.

In the present study, during the early years of marriage, the female respondents reported that their family members and relatives were more loving, cooperative and understanding; but as the problem was diagnosed, they observed a change in their relationship. It was reported by female respondents that their family members had become quarrelsome, frustrated over small matters and husband had increased alcohol intake and used to stay out of home for a comparatively increased duration. In some cases they avoided their wife's company.

Gender difference was seen in the fact that the respondents found it easier to put the blame on women. Men's infertility was generally kept as a secret. The wives themselves actively helped to keep it a secret when husbands were diagnosed infertile.

> Childless couples are under social and religious pressures that compel them to continuously try various methods for procreation as it is the offspring who is responsible for the continuation of the family line.

With the help of various government organisations and NGOs, allopathic treatment has spread to most of the villages, and with the help of health camps, satellite hospitals, primary health centres, etc., the people have been educated about all the latest diseases, their symptoms and their cures. Yet their faith in alternative therapy is not shaken.

Along with medical treatment, respondents try non-medical treatment that includes consulting astrologers, saints, magico-spiritual healers, Reiki clinics, visiting various shrines, following religious practices, etc. To the extent that their domestic chores allowed, women performed regular prayers and chanted passages from holy books either at home or at places of worship. They undertook fasts in honour of specific gods, eating or avoiding certain foods on specific days. On Fridays, for example, they might honour the goddess Santoshi Mata by eating only once and avoiding sour items in their food.

When questioned about the replacement of man or woman for a fixed tenure, nearly all the couples said that this kind of practice is only possible in the western countries and will be considered as a sin in the Indian society.

But many couples including those who have had love marriage are generally perturbed due to childlessness and so more than a third of such couples are ready to use any means. Couples, who had arranged marriages, would decide to undergo recognised treatments or for test-tube babies.

Any scientific or modern method is considered as an alternative, which is not necessarily accepted by family or society, but can give a child. During this study, many incidences are found to explore the secrets, which are more likely to be unethical in Indian society.

Doctors themselves said that they did it with their patient's consent and childless couples also agreed upon this that they are confident about their confidentiality. The childless couples need a child so badly that they agreed to do anything whether ethical or not, to get a child.

> Sterility and infertility rank high as the most difficult reproductive problems. Besides being and handled as a medical problem, these have personal, psychological, social and cultural aspects.

For couples that discover that they cannot have children for whatever reason, the loss of parenthood, a basic ingredient of life, comes as a rude shock.

Childless couples often focus their attention on failure and when this is done, they undergo different types of losses, i.e., loss of relationship, loss of health, loss of status or prestige, loss of self-esteem, loss of self-confidence, loss of security, loss of fantasy and loss of something or someone of great symbolic value.

Loss of significant relationship is an unspoken fear. Because both the man and woman are hurting, tired and under great pressure they feel depleted of physical and emotional energy. They may become less able to fulfil each other's need and thereby suffer a loss of closeness to the point of feeling worlds apart.

> Even after so much of medical advancement and awareness, the importance of religious practices also coexist.

Many respondents believe that medical treatment works only, if one had good luck and if God wanted to give a child to someone. Respondents who are already religious, become more religious and those who are not religious start believing in God. They keep fasts, attend religious ceremonies, and visit holy shrines, pilgrimage, and even start taking bath on special occasions.

Astrologers recommend fasting on particular days for a particular period to time according to the stars of couples. Suggestions are given on the basis of horoscopes of the couples. Particular gems are also suggested for wearing on fingers. Various modes of *pujas* (worship) are suggested. Religious books are recommended for studying. In general, women were more meticulous in their performance of these rituals than were men. Often, by keeping them occupied, the rituals were helpful as coping strategies for living with infertility.

> Males are more hesitant in seeking medical assistance and treatment for childlessness as compared to females.

It is clear that men are hesitant to get their potency tested. In some cases husbands do not wish to get themselves examined first for childlessness and some of the husbands never went to medical examination although they were worried about the problem. In order to keep their tests a secret and due to the social and economic status, more than 40 per cent of the urban men, choose to bear the excessive amount of expenses and get themselves checked-up in private clinics.

More behavioural changes found in females because of childlessness as compared to the males.

There is a difference in the behaviour of men and women. On being invited to a child's birthday party, the attitude of men ranges from that of happiness to normalcy. Similarly, on seeing a pregnant woman or on looking at the toys and clothes of children, their behaviour does not become tense, even when they themselves are responsible for childlessness. On the contrary, women feel tense on attending a child's birthday party and the same feeling arises when they see a pregnant woman. A great difference in the behaviour of men and women has been observed when they see a child of their relatives or on being invited to any special occasion.

On seeing a relative's child, men feel happy; on the other hand, women consider themselves inferior and feel separated and they hesitate to socialise on such occasions and so develop tensions.

SOCIO-ECONOMIC FACTORS AFFECTING CHILDLESS COUPLES

The analysis of socio-economic profile of childless couples (Table 7.1) indicates major differences in the marital life and family situations. Varied experiences are reported in social interactions and behaviour. Medical assistance and treatment included traditional beliefs and alternative therapies. Most of the couples consulted traditional healers before medical examination. Modes of tension management are: service, religious participation, household work, education and adoption.

To analyse the research problem, four institutional factors, i.e., caste, family, duration of marriage, and type of marriage are taken as background characteristics. Two demographic factors, age of husband and age of wife are also covered in the profile. For assessing standard of living, the characteristics

Table 7.1
Socio-Economic Factors Affecting Childless Couples

Characteristics	*Marital Life and Family Situations*	*Social Interactions and Behaviour*	*Medical Assistance and Treatment*	*Tension Management Processes*
Residence (Rural, Urban slums, Urban)	***	**	***	*
House (Kachcha, Semi-pucca, Pucca)	***	*	**	*
Wife's Age (19 to 40+ years)	***	*	***	***
Husband's Age (19 to 40+ years)	**	*	**	*
Duration of Marriage (Less than 3 to 18+ years)	*	***	**	**
Caste (General, SC, ST, OBC)	**	**	***	*
Family (Nuclear, Joint)		**	*	*
Husband's Occupation (Business, Service, Agriculture)	***	***	**	**
Wife's Occupation (Business, Service, Agriculture, Housewife)	***	**	**	**
Monthly Income (Less than Rs. 2000 to 8000+)	**	**	**	*
Type of Marriage (Love marriage, Arranged marriage)	*	**	*	

* To little extent; ** To some extent; *** To great extent.

residence, house, occupation, and income have been included (Table 7.1). Residence (rural, urban slums, urban) greatly affects marital life and family situation, social interaction and behaviour, medical assistance and treatment. More problems are identified for the childless couples in urban slums. However, the residential environment has little effect on tension management processes of the couples. Similarly, the nature of house greatly influences the marital life and medical treatment aspects. The problems are comparatively severe in couples residing in semi-*pucca* houses. Rural women were more eager for treatment because they experienced greater social pressure from the community. It has been observed that caste and practice of alternative therapies are deeply linked with each other. The use of witchcraft has been greater among Scheduled Tribes (STs). The period of marriage affects the uses of alternatives. After long duration of married life childless couples are prepared to use some modern means like test-tube baby. Coping mechanisms are more frequently adopted by females when hope of conception ends. Age of wife and husband differentiates marital life and family situations and medical treatment of the couples. Age of wife greatly affects the tension management processes. Family life situations appeared to change little because of the duration of marriage.

Caste reveals some impact on marital life, family and social interaction; having some effect on medical treatment and a little effect on management of couples' tensions. The problems are comparatively more in scheduled and other backward classes, where caste factor appears to exercise greater effect.

Type of family has some effect on social interactions but little effect on medical treatment and tension management and no effect on marital life. But husband's and wife's occupations have greater influence on the social life of childless couples. This is also true in case of the monthly income of the couples. The duration of marriage has great impact on social interactions.

SOCIAL, INSTITUTIONAL AND BEHAVIOURAL DIMENSIONS

There is no significant change in the social and institutional dimensions of childless couples in the Indian society. Although behavioural modifications have been noticed because of the change in standard of living of the childless couples, inability to produce a child is considered more of a social stigma than physical disability. The institutional dimension is prominently determined by the caste considerations and duration of marital life. Occupations, place of residence and type of house, which are linked to the standard of living, bring in behavioural modifications in marital life and family situation. Rural, slum or urban living determines the mode of medical treatment. Social conflict and avoidance is more prominent in urban slums (Table 4.1) and *kachcha* house (Table 4.4), which are related to level of dissatisfaction in the married life. Social interactions and behaviours of couples are associated to their occupations. When the couple is engaged in agriculture, their marital life and social interactions are greatly affected by childlessness (Table 4.8).

If the couples are in service, they undergo better and longer medical treatment for tension management. All the aspects of standard of living are covered in behavioural dimension because they reduce the dissatisfaction of couples, but do not necessarily increase the level of satisfaction. Here 'dissatisfaction' and 'satisfaction' are considered as two separate dimensions; dissatisfaction as a contributor of the standard of living associated with the behavioural modification. This does not increase the satisfaction or 'happiness at heart' but only changes the behavioural aspects 'overt happiness'. The support from the caste and change in the interaction modes of caste traditions favouring childless couples can add to their level of real satisfaction. Age of wife, which is a demographic variable, has a social institutional significance also. Women maintain traditions and accept established patterns as fait accompli during childlessness. As the age increases, they naturalise social interactions in their community. The age of husband has some effect on the marital life and medical assistance but it is the women who suffer more and for a longer period than their husbands. The behavioural aspects are more of coping mechanism associated to the standard of living.

The factors which greatly affect social consequences of childlessness are social institutional, or impact-oriented whereas the behavioural factors are effect-oriented. Social

Figure 7.1

Social, Institutional and Behavioural Dimensions in Childlessness

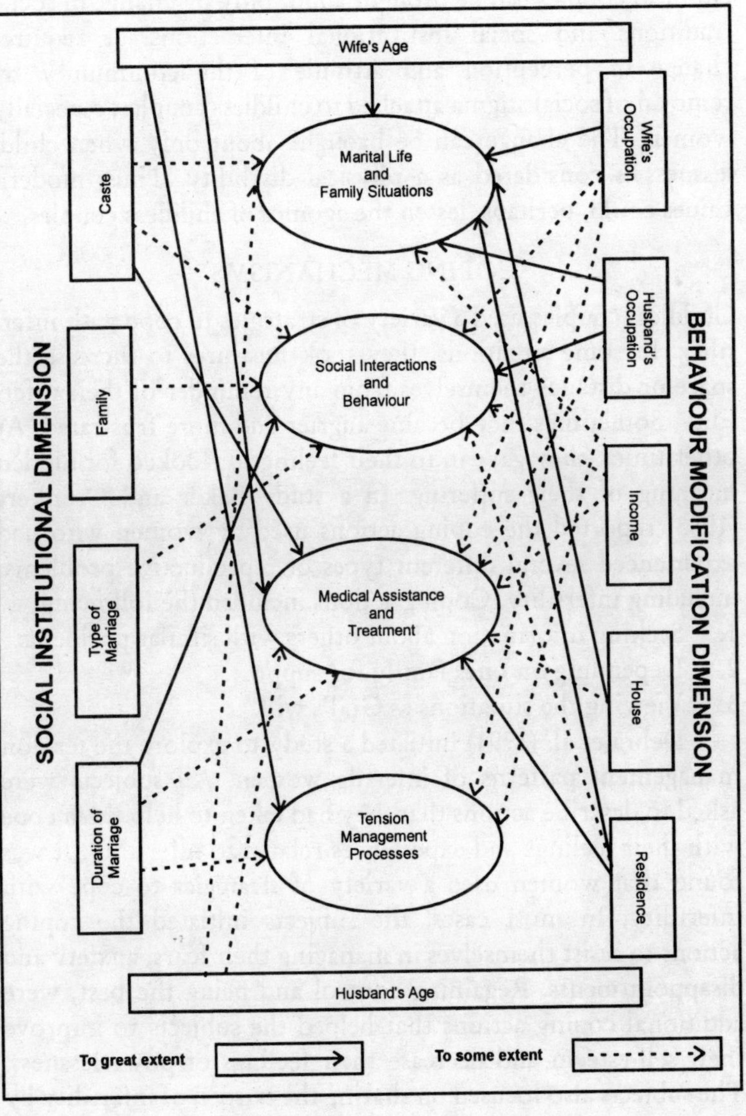

impact is a long-term phenomenon whereas the effect, which is behavioural is short lived, temporary and varying according to the standard of living. The impact change in the life of the childless couples can be brought about only by change in social traditions and social institutional interactions. It requires change in perception and attitude of the community by removal of social stigma attached to childless couples, especially women. The change can be brought about only when childlessness is considered as a physical disability. Thus, modern values could, perhaps, lessen the agonies of childless couples.

COPING MECHANISMS

Childless couples used a variety of strategies to cope with infertility. In some situations, they took measures to increase the space or distance themselves from any reminder of their infertility. Sometimes they became angrier and more frustrated. At other times, they gave in to their feelings or looked for hidden meaning of their suffering. In a study Baker and Quinkert (1983) reported the coping actions used by women who had experienced several different types of reproductive problems, including infertility. Coping actions included the following:

1. Seeking information about others with similar problems.
2. Depending on ones family for support.
3. Viewing the situations as God's will.

Debra et al. (1991) initiated a study to explore the tension management patterns of infertile women. All subjects were asked to describe actions that they had taken to help them cope with their feelings and experiences related to infertility. It was found that women used a variety of strategies to cope with infertility. In most cases, the subjects initiated the coping actions to assist themselves in managing their fears, anxiety and disappointments. Regaining control and being the best, were additional coping actions that helped the subjects to improve their self-esteem and decrease their feelings of powerlessness. The subjects also focused on sharing the burden of infertility by sharing their feelings and experiences with others. The women reported that sharing their feelings and concerns with husbands, friends, relatives and especially other infertile couples proved helpful. Unfortunately none of the subject stated that health care providers helped them to manage tensions. Deodar (1995) studied the coping patterns and activities adopted by the childless couples. It was found that majority of the respondents noticed a change in their behaviour and personality. Most of the women felt that keeping themselves occupied through jobs, hobby activities and work helped them to cope with infertility. Majority of the respondents was aware of different forms of treatment for childlessness and they expressed a high hope in the success of medical treatment. For most of the respondents, child adoption was a lesser-preferred alternative in comparison to the treatment. Some respondents were aware of the opinion that they would never opt for child adoption

According to this study, those respondents, who were positive towards life, more frequently adopted coping patterns. A few couples understood the broader meaning of life and compromised with the situation. They made themselves busy in other activities. They were of the opinion that they would not want to waste their whole life in frustration and depression but they wanted to make best use of their lives. Some of them kept themselves busy with the children of neighbours, relatives, and friends or of extended family members. Some others had joined social service.

Many of the respondents turned towards religion to cope up with the situation of childlessness. They started believing in religion and started performing religious activities like praying, going on pilgrimage, and performing rituals, reading religious books. Those couples who had positive attitude towards the problem of infertility were found to be well adjusted in their families, workplaces and society and those who had negative attitude towards the problem were found to be maladjusted. Some respondents reported that their relations did not suffer because of infertility but had become stronger. There was no friction due to childlessness. More positive interpersonal relations were also reported. Respondents stated that more love and affection developed between the couple and their relationship faced no threat as the bond between them was strong and they used to support and console each other by saying:

> Nobody can be blamed in this matter. It is the wish of God.

It was found that some couples often tried to approach other people's children, especially those who belonged to his family; and they had a favourable attitude to other people's children and they liked being in their company. Some of the respondents also had positive feelings towards pregnancy of others and they consider them as lucky because they are complete and they will not face the psychosocial repercussions of childlessness. They felt happy about pregnancy of others. After waiting for a long time to have a child, daily routine of childless couples undergo changes. More participation in religious activities has seen a rise among males. They take more interest in social activities and perform acts of social well-being in many ways. Due to childlessness, affectionate behaviour towards orphan has been found mostly in men. Women, comparatively, take more interest in contributing clothes, medicines and food, etc., to charitable organisation. Men spend money for social causes with a free-hand whereas women do hold religious feelings, sympathy and pity in their hearts but hesitate to spend money for this.

It was also found that parents having a positive and sympathetic attitude towards the problem faced by childless couples. Respondents stated that they were understanding and cooperative. They understood the couple and their feelings very well and tried to avoid such circumstances, which could hurt their feelings. They neither made demands on the couple to bear a child, nor criticised the behaviour of the affected couple. Whenever the affected couple got depressed or felt isolated, they tried to console and encourage by saying such words as:

> "Have faith in God", "God will help you one day", "Believe in God, everything will be alright."

On the basis of this study, it is suggested that childlessness deserves serious attention and should be considered as a physical disability. It would be better if this problem is viewed integrating the various dimensions of the issue, by getting the doctors, family members, relatives and society into the picture.

The childless couples can also opt for new reproductive techniques, i.e., Non-Coital Reproductive Techniques (NCRTs). They are popularly known as 'test-tube baby techniques' and used for treating certain types of childlessness. Presently, *In Vitro* Fertilization-Embryo Transfer (IVF-ET) and Gamete Intra-Fallopian Transfer (GIFT) are used in India.

The psychosomatic aspect of childlessness still has the utmost validity. Balancing the wish for child, in the context of all other life wishes can set the stage for a couple-community relationship. Counselling of childless couples helps in minimising tension and provides a better life. Trained counsellors could be more helpful in reducing the negative effects of childlessness without disclosing their identity.

It would be worthwhile to arrange training programmes for the couples to help them in understanding their body mechanisms and prevent unhealthy practises, which may result in childlessness. Lack of awareness of the main causes of childlessness leads to many negative impacts on childless couples. Educational programmes would help to solve many of these problems. In general hospitals also, specialised infertility clinics for investigation and treatment need to be developed. Because, childlessness is not just a "woman's disease", both of the partners should get their status of fertility checked.

Active coping mechanisms could be adopted by couples who have positive attitude and want to make best use of their lives. They should not waste their whole life in waiting for a child when it is not possible. Most of the women felt that keeping themselves occupied through jobs, hobby activities, and work helped them to cope with infertility. They should go outside and interact not only in limited social circles but make wider circle beyond caste level activities. They can take more interest in social activities and perform acts of social well-being in many ways. To fill the vacuum of their life, for continuation of family lineage, adoption as an alternative can be also used.

References

Baker, M.A. and Quinkert, A. (1983). Women's Reactions to Reproductive Problems. Psycho Report.

Berger, D. and David (1980). Psychological Assessment of the Infertile Couples. *American Journal of Psychiatry.*

Billimoria, H.M. (1984). *Child Adoption: A Study of Indian Experience.* Himalayan Publications, Mumbai.

Freedman, R. and Whelpton Campbell (1959). *Family Planning: Sterility and Population Growth.* McGraw Hill Book Company Inc.

Harrison, M. (1964). *A Couple's Guide to Cause and Treatments.* Houghton Mifflin Company, Boston.

Inhorn, M.C. (1994). Interpreting Infertility: Medical Anthropological Perspective, Introduction. *Social Science and Medicine.*

Insler, V. (1981). *Some Epidemiological Aspects of Fertility Evaluation.* Elsevier North Holland, New York.

Jacobson and Lalos, A. (1986). A Psychosocial Characterisation of Infertile Couples before Surgical Treatment of the Female. *Journal of Psychosomatic Obstetrics and Gynecology.*

Lalos, A. et al. (1985). The Wish to Have a Child: A Pilot Study of the Infertile Couples. *Acta Psychiatrica Scandinavica.*

Mandelbaum, David G. (1970). *Society in India.* University of California Press, Berkeley.

Masters, W.H. and Johnson, V.E. (1970). *Human Sexual Inadequacy.* Little Brown, Boston.

Mathur, Neeta (1989). *A Psychological Study of Infertile Women.* Ph.D. thesis in Psychology. Mohan Lal Sukhadia University, Udaipur.

Renne, K.S. (1977). Childlessness, Health and Marital Satisfaction. Social Biology.

Rosenfeld (1985). The Psychosocial Component of Infertility. *Journal of Fertility and Sterility.*

Shapiro, D.H. and Constance, H. (1982). The Impact of Infertility on the Marital Relationship. *Social Casework.*

Sharma, S.P. (1990). Childlessness: Bane or Boon. *Women's Era*. July (second).

Sheshadri, A. (1990). *Perception of Childless Couples Regarding Childlessness, Treatment and Adoption.* Project report submitted to Tata Institute of Social Science, Mumbai.

Stewart, S., and Glazer, G. (1986). Expectations and Coping of Women Undergoing *In Vitro* Fertilization. *Maternity Child Nursing Journal,* 15(2).

Bibliography

Abbey, A., Andrew, F.M. and Halman, L.J. (1991). The Importance of Social Relationship for Infertile Couples Well-being. In Al. Stanton and C. Dunkeescheltes (eds.), *Psychological Adjustment to Infertility*, Plenum, New York.

Abdullah, A. and Zeidenstein, D. (1982). *Rites and Ceremonies of Hindus and Muslims.* Amar Prakashan, Delhi.

Abse, D. (1966). Psychiatric Aspects of Human Male Infertility. *American Journal of Fertility and Sterility*, 17.

Ahmed, A. (1991). *Women and Fertility in Bangladesh.* Sage Publications, New Delhi.

Anand, U. (1984). Infertility and Infertility Counselling. *Journal of Family Welfare*, 31(2).

Bennett, F.J. (1965). The Social, Cultural and Emotional Aspects of Sterility in Women in Buganda. *Journal of Fertility and Sterility*, *16.*

Brand, H.J. (1981). The Influence of Sex Difference on the Acceptance of Infertility. *South African Journal of Psychology*, 11(4).

Brand, J. and Roos, S.S. (1982). Psychological Stress and Infertility: Psychophysiological Patterns. *British Journal of Medical Psychology*, 55(4).

Butterworth's Medical Dictionary (1990). Butterworth & Co. (Publishers) Limited English Language Book Society.

Campbell, F.L., Towner, B.D. and Beach, L.R. (1982). Cited by Diana E. Papila and Salley Wandkos, *Human Development* (3rd Edition), Tata McGraw Hill Publication Inc. Pvt. Ltd., New Delhi.

Churchill's Medical Dictionary (1981). Churchill Livingstone, New York, Edinburgh, London, Melbourne.

Collin's Concise Encyclopedia (1984). Peerage Books, London.

Danieli, I.D. (1982). Childless and Marital Adjustment in Northern Nigeria. *Journal of Marriage and the Family Adjustment*, 44.

Davis K. and Blake J. (1956). *Economic Development and Social Change.* Social Structure and Fertility, an Analytic Framework. Vol. 4.

Deodar, S.C. (1995). *Infertility and Adoption Option.* Unpublished project report submitted to Tata Institute of Social Science (TISS), Mumbai.

Dixit, D. (1991). *Childless Couples.* Social Welfare, 37.

Dubin, A. and Lawrence (1972). *Sexual Causes of Male Infertility.* Excerpta Medica, 18.

Frank, (1994). Infertility and Subjective Well-being. The Mediating Role of Self-esteem, Internal Control and Interpersonal Conflict. *Journal of Marriage and the Family*, 32.

Freedman, R. (1963). *The Sociology of Human Fertility.* A trend report and bibliography, Basil Blackwell, Oxford.

Gupta, L. and Shrivastava, D. (1982). Infertile Couples and Neuroticism. *Indian Journal of Clinical Psychology*, 9(1).

Harrison, M. (1964). *Infertility a Couple's Guide to Causes and Treatments.* Houghton Mifflin Company, Boston, 10.

Hoffman, L.W. (1988). Cross Cultural Differences in Child Rearing Goals. In R.A. Levin, P.M. Miller and M.M. West (eds.) *Parental Behaviour in Diverse Societies.* Jossey Bass, San Francisco.

Hull and Valerie, J. (1980). *Intermediate Variables in the Explanation of Differential Fertility: Results of a Village in Rural Java.* Human Ecology, 8(3).

Inhorn, M.C. (1994). *Interpreting Infertility: Medical Anthropological Perspectives.* Social Science and Medicine (Elmsford, New York) Vol. 39, No.4 (August).

Jacobson and Lalos, A. (1986). A Psychosocial Characterization of Infertile Couples Before Surgical Treatment of the Female. *Journal of Psychosomatic Obstetrics and Gynecology*, 4(2).

Lalos, A. et al. (1985). *The Wish to Have a Child: A Pilot Study of the Infertile Couples.* Acta Psychiatrica Scandinavica, 72(5).

Malpani, A. and Chuna, B. (1995). *Getting Pregnant: A Guide for Infertile Couples.* USB Publishing Ltd., New Delhi.

Mann, K. (1996). *Tribal Women on the Threshold of 21st Century.* M.D. Publications, New Delhi.

Master, W.H. and Johnson, V.E. (1970). *Human Sexual Inadequacy.* Little Brown, Boston.

Mathews, A.N. and Mathews, R. (1986). Beyond the Mechanics of Infertility: Perspectives on Social Psychology of Infertility and Voluntary Childlessness. *Family Relations.* 35(4).

Mathur, Neeta (1989). *A Psychological Study of Infertile Married Women.* Ph.D. thesis in Psychology, M.L. Sukhadia University.

Miall, C.E. (1994). *Community Construct of Involuntary Childlessness: Sympathy, Stigma and Social Support.* Canadian Review of Sociology and Anthropology. Sociology and Anthropology, 31(4).

Mishell, D. Davajan (1991). *Evaluation of the Infertile Couple.* Infertility, Contraception and Reproductive Endocrinology, Blackwell Scientific 557, Boston.

Mulgaonkar, V.B. (2001). Childless Couples in the Slums of Mumbai: An Interdisciplinary Study. *Asia-Pacific Population Journal,* June.

Patel, T. (1994). *Fertility Behaviour, Population and Society in a Rajasthan Village.* Oxford University Press, Delhi.

Rahman, O. and Jane Menken (1993). Age at Menopause and Fecundity Preceeding Menopause. *Biomedical and Demographic Determinants of Reproduction*, Ronald Gray, Henri Leridon and Alfred Spria (eds.) Clarendon Press, Oxford.

Reddy and Mahadevan (1986). Certain Correlates of Conformity. Child Psychitary.

Sharma, P.C. et al. (1970). Etiological Correlates of Family Divorce Rates Due to Sterility. *Journal of Family Welfare*, 17(2).

Sharma, S.P. (1990). Childlessness: Bane or Boon. *Women's Era*, 26, July (Second).

Upadhyay, Chakrapani (2001). *Socio-Cultural and Demographic Determinants of Reproductive Health: A Study of Tribes of Southern Rajasthan.* Ph.D. thesis, M.L. Sukhadia University, Udaipur.

Vaessan, M. (1984). *Childlessness and Infecundity,* Comparative Study, 31, London World Fertility Survey.

World Health Organisation (1991). *Programme on Maternal and Child Health and Family Planning.* Division of Family Health. Infertility: A Tabulation of Available Data on Prevalence of Primary and Secondary Infertility, WHO/MCH/91-9, World Health Organisation, Geneva.

World Health Organisation (1991). *Challenges in Reproductive Health Research: Biannual Report.* World Health Organisation, Geneva.

WEBSITES ON CHILDLESSNESS

http://www.who.int/reproductive-health/infertility/ii.pdf

http://www.vedalink.com/children.htm

http://www.hsph.harvard.edu/organizations/healthnet/sasia/suchana/0225/jejeebhoy.htm

http://www.whosea.org/women/ch3-4.htm

http://www.pofsupport.org/newsletters/july2001f.htm

http://www.apa.org/monitor/jan01/parenthood.html

http://www.unescap.org/pop/journal/2001/v16n2a9.pdf

http://www.indiainformation.com/health/resources.htm

http://www.who.int/reproductive-health/new/news57.pdf

http://www.tribuneindia.com/2001/20010116/main8.htm

http://www.popcouncil.org/pdfs/menaspartners.pdf

http://www.ourworld.compuserve.com/homepages/johnflanagan/wb-paber-perri.doc

Index